Understanding and Enhancing Positive Regard in Psychotherapy

Under one cover this book offers a rich and thorough review of the history and philosophical roots of positive regard (PR), the related empirical research, and a practical guide for clinical uses. It provides both an "inside" (within the client-centered) and broader pantheoretical perspective. The authors offer a deep appreciation of the value of PR and, at the same time, also carefully delineate the limits and challenges associated with the concept. This outstanding book is a rare combination of scientific rigor and tried clinical wisdom in an accessible and engaging format—an essential item in the library of every psychologist.

—**Adam O. Horvath, EdD,** Professor Emeritus, Simon Fraser University, Past President of Society for Psychotherapy Research, North American Chapter

A very important book. There never has been as thorough a treatment of positive regard as there is in this book. It gets at the research, and it does a thorough review of its history, theoretical notions, and clinical use. I recommend it for practitioners, theorists, teachers, and researchers. Finally, it is readable and interesting. Even Carl Rogers's alter ego, Mr. Rogers, makes an appearance!

—**Arthur C. Bohart, PhD,** Professor Emeritus, California State University, Dominguez Hills

The positive regard that these authors have for their readers, clients, students, and colleagues is apparent. This well-written book will help readers think about the role that a therapist's authenticity and well-being play in their work with clients. I recommend it to everyone who wants to become a better person and a better therapist.

—**Clara E. Hill, PhD,** Professor, University of Maryland, College Park

Understanding and Enhancing Positive Regard in Psychotherapy

CARL ROGERS AND BEYOND

Barry A. Farber, Jessica Y. Suzuki, and Daisy Ort

AMERICAN PSYCHOLOGICAL ASSOCIATION

Published by
American Psychological Association
750 First Street, NE
Washington, DC 20002
https://www.apa.org

Order Department
https://www.apa.org/pubs/books
order@apa.org

In the U.K., Europe, Africa, and the Middle East, copies may be ordered from Eurospan
https://www.eurospanbookstore.com/apa
info@eurospangroup.com

Typeset in Charter and Interstate by Circle Graphics, Inc., Reisterstown, MD

Printer: Gasch Printing, Odenton, MD
Cover Designer: Schlenoff Design, Bethesda, MD

Library of Congress Cataloging-in-Publication Data

Names: Farber, Barry A. (Barry Alan), 1947- author. | Suzuki, Jessica Y., author. | Ort, Daisy, author.
Title: Understanding and enhancing positive regard in psychotherapy : Carl Rogers and beyond / by Barry A. Farber, Jessica Y. Suzuki, and Daisy Ort.
Description: Washington, DC : American Psychological Association, [2022] | Includes bibliographical references and index.
Identifiers: LCCN 2022008521 (print) | LCCN 2022008522 (ebook) | ISBN 9781433836695 (paperback) | ISBN 9781433840715 (ebook)
Subjects: LCSH: Rogers, Carl R. (Carl Ransom), 1902–1987. | Client-centered psychotherapy. | BISAC: PSYCHOLOGY / Psychotherapy / General | PSYCHOLOGY / Clinical Psychology
Classification: LCC RC481 .F37 2022 (print) | LCC RC481 (ebook) | DDC 616.89/14--dc23/eng/20220318
LC record available at https://lccn.loc.gov/2022008521
LC ebook record available at https://lccn.loc.gov/2022008522

https://doi.org/10.1037/0000312-000

Printed in the United States of America

10 9 8 7 6 5 4 3 2 1

To those for whom I have felt unconditional positive regard and love and to those whose positive regard for me has felt so loving: Laurie; Alissa and Dan; David and Genna; Ava, Avi, Zoe, and Elliott; Neal and Varda; Wayne and Jean; Spears and Kayla; Jillian and Andrew; and Ian.

— BARRY A. FARBER

For Rocket, River, and Tom. I am the LUCKIEST.

— JESSICA Y. SUZUKI

To mom: For loving me unconditionally "to infinity and back." To Tom: You are a gem.

— DAISY ORT

Contents

Acknowledgments

We would like to acknowledge the extremely helpful assistance of the many graduate students at Teachers College, Columbia University, who have been committed members of our research team over these past years and contributed greatly to the literature reviews and research noted in this book, including (in alphabetical order): Dina Alghabra, Jenna Cohen, Rachel Floyd, Yifan Gao, Jacob Hermann, Emily Hubbard, Yinan Liang, Shibo Lyu, Katherine Donatela Manlongat, Lauren McMullen, Tanya Mehdizadeh, Lauren O'Leary, Emily Pfannenstiel, Will Runge, Paula Ryszkiewicz, Mingrui Wu, and Meltem Yilmaz. Special shout-outs to Gus Mayopoulos (who co-led the Positive Regard lab for a year and contributed significantly to the section in this book about the role of positive regard in social media) and to Caitlin Moore (a member of our research team who compiled and edited multiple versions of the References section). We also extend our sincere appreciation to two very talented, recently graduated doctoral students in our program, David Lynch and Amar Mandavia, for their help with the statistical analyses of some of our previously published papers on positive regard.

We also greatly appreciate the comments, suggestions, and feedback on earlier drafts of this book of many extremely wise and thoughtful colleagues, including (in alphabetical order) Godfrey T. Barrett-Lennard, Art Bohart, David Cain, Jesse Geller, George Goldstein, Adam Horvath, Dale Larson, Germain Lietaer, Sam Menahem, David Roe, and Kirk Schneider. Their input has been invaluable.

Understanding and Enhancing Positive Regard in Psychotherapy

INTRODUCTION

MEETING CARL ROGERS

I (BAF) met Carl Rogers only briefly. It was in 1986, a year before he died, and as a newly tenured faculty member in the clinical psychology program at Teachers College, Columbia University—Rogers's alma mater—I was given the honor of hosting him for 2 days when he was awarded the college's Medal of Honor. "Hosting" consisted mostly of picking him up at his hotel a couple of miles from the college and driving him back at the conclusion of both his days—one spent primarily meeting with senior faculty, college officials, and important donors, the other at the college's graduation ceremonies. Nevertheless, I did get to have some private conversations with him, and these turned out to have a significant impact on my career.

I have a fatherly image of Carl Rogers and a cherished picture of the two of us in my academic office, but what I remember most was the quality of his listening. His was a serious, attentive, nonbantering type of listening—one I was not accustomed to. It had a psychotherapeutic quality but absent the need for psychoanalytic inquiry. He seemed genuinely interested in my career and answered

https://doi.org/10.1037/0000312-001
Understanding and Enhancing Positive Regard in Psychotherapy: Carl Rogers and Beyond, by B. A. Farber, J. Y. Suzuki, and D. Ort

my questions with a great deal of consideration and earnestness. A case in point: At that time, I was studying stress and burnout in teachers and psychotherapists and asked him, while driving him back to his hotel that first day, whether he had ever felt burned out. Dr. Rogers—and that is what I called him at that point—thought for a moment and then replied, "Let me think about that and get back to you about that." Nearly all the time, a reply like that essentially means, "I'm not particularly interested in that question, let's talk about something else." When I picked him up at his hotel the next morning, almost immediately following quick pleasantries, he said to me something on the order of, "I've been thinking about that question you asked me yesterday. I really haven't felt burned out doing counseling. I have occasionally felt frustrated but not to the point where I wanted to stop doing the work or felt exhausted by it." It wasn't the content of his answer that surprised me. It was the fact that he had apparently thought seriously about what I had asked the day before and treated my question with such a great deal of respect. I do not think he was fascinated by the question—to my knowledge, Carl Rogers never wrote about the vocational hazards or potential for burnout in his work—but his way of being in the world, his sense of what it means to be a person, mandated that he treat me respectfully, caringly, even appreciatively. (Subsequent to his visit, he wrote me a very gracious handwritten letter that I still have framed in my office.)

Was I in awe of this quite-famous person—surely the most famous psychologist of his time—and did this affect my perceptions of our encounter? Yes, of course. But at the time of our meeting, I was far more knowledgeable about, and a believer in, both psychodynamic theory (the predominant therapeutic orientation of my doctoral program at Yale a few years earlier) and even behavioral therapies (what I had learned when I was a special education teacher prior to graduate school, the topic of my first professional publication, and what I was then teaching at Teachers College). I was not especially inclined to learn more about his theories or be influenced professionally by meeting Carl Rogers. I was looking forward deeply to meeting this extraordinarily influential man, especially as he was instrumental in advancing the human potential movement of the late 60s that, as a college student at the time, I was somewhat touched by. But, like many in the field—shamefully, far too many—I had an image of him and his theories as neither deep enough (per conventional psychoanalytic thinking) nor concerned enough with directly effecting change (per conventional behavioral and cognitive behavioral thinking).

I did not come away from my time with Carl Rogers a "true believer"—that is, as an advocate for the position that client-centered therapy was the best or even preferred way to do clinical work or that Rogers's three core therapist-provided attitudes (empathy, positive regard [PR], genuineness) were the necessary and sufficient factors in therapeutic change. In fact, I later wrote an article (Farber, 2007) arguing that although his conditions had an enduring and substantial influence on the field, especially in arguing for the critical importance of the therapy relationship per se, they were "not-quite necessary nor sufficient" (p. 289).

And yet. Primarily as a result of my meeting Carl Rogers, I became and remain intrigued by his way of doing therapy—indeed, his way of being with people—especially the integral role of conveying to others a sense of PR. He made those with whom he spoke feel important through active listening, empathic statements, attempts to check his understanding, and sustained eye contact. Though it's somewhat of an oxymoron, Carl Rogers struck me as both low-key and highly charismatic. I wanted to learn more about this man and his iconoclastic views on what clients need from their psychotherapists. I began this part of my career, my Rogers portion, by coediting, with two colleagues at the time—Patricia Raskin at Teachers College and Debora Brink, a retired faculty member at City College and a close friend of Carl's— a (1996) book about his clinical cases, *The Psychotherapy of Carl Rogers: Cases and Commentary*. We transcribed or summarized 10 of Rogers's cases and asked clinicians from both inside and outside the person-centered community to comment on his work. Some chose to comment quite favorably on his approach, noting that his consistent adherence to his theoretical propositions led to a successful clinical encounter. But many commentators, including some who identified with the client- or person-centered approach, found much to be wanting, noting, among things, that Rogers was more directive, explicitly affirming, and interpretive than his writings would suggest; that he was naïve to gender, sexual, and cultural issues within the relationship; and that he avoided acknowledging negative feelings (Farber et al., 1996).

That he was not perfect, nor even perfectly consistent with his own theoretical model, was neither surprising nor disappointing. No founder of any major theoretical system has managed to hew precisely to the principles they have proposed. People are just too variable and their needs too protean. Wise therapists understand that. But if Rogers was not consistently nondirective, he was consistently supportive, caring, and positively regarding. That was what came through in the commentaries in the book as well as in the demonstration videos Rogers participated in. That was intriguing. Furthermore, whereas at that time (late 1990s) there had already been a good deal of research on the nature and impact of therapist-provided empathy and even a fair amount of theoretical and clinical literature on the role of therapist genuineness, comparatively little written had been about PR. There were some summaries of the effects of PR (often under the classification of "therapist affirmation"), most notably in the influential psychotherapy research series *Bergin and Garfield's*

Handbook of Psychotherapy and Behavior Change (1971, 1993). But there was an absence of studies on how PR actually manifests in psychotherapy. If it was, as Rogers thought, an attitude, how was that attitude conveyed? What were the behavioral markers? Did clients and therapists differ in the ways they perceived the nature and consequences of PR? What client, therapist, and treatment variables are associated with differences in perceptions of what types of PR are most often provided in therapy, and what types are experienced as most affirming?

THE ELEMENTS OF THIS BOOK

Investigating the myriad ways in which Rogers and other clinicians could convey PR, the variables affecting its perceived intensity and frequency of occurrence and its association to therapeutic outcome became the focus of our Positive Regard lab at Teachers College. We—myself and a host of doctoral- and master's-level psychology students participating in the lab—were interested in finding multiple ways of exploring these topics: case studies, interviews with clients and therapists, development of new assessment instruments to measure PR, survey research, and meta-analyses. Two extremely talented clinical psychology doctoral students who led these labs are the coauthors of this book: Jessi Suzuki, a recent (2018) graduate, and Daisy Ort, a soon-to-be graduate of the program.

In one sense, then, this book represents the next logical step in the sequence of our investigations of PR: synthesizing in one volume the studies our lab and others have conducted on this topic in recent years and augmenting this empirical focus with case examples. In another sense, this book seems particularly appropriate now—a time when there seems to be a paucity of goodwill and acceptance of others in the world, a time when a consideration of the ways in which PR can be conveyed in the clinical realm and beyond might be a meaningful professional contribution. It is in this second sense that *Carl Rogers and Beyond* serves as the subtitle of this book, a reflection of the awareness that a book about PR in these times should include discussion of the way that this attitude of relating to others has been manifest in clinical orientations other than person-centered therapy (albeit under different terms) and, importantly, extend beyond the psychotherapeutic setting. Rogers was aware of the value of applying his approach to nonclinical situations, working in the later years of his life with individuals looking to further their self-awareness through encounter groups and with activists in highly toxic political arenas around the world. In this book, we take our inspiration from Rogers and note the ways that nonclinicians have modeled PR in their lives and look, too, at the ways in which PR is conveyed through social media.

We begin this book (Chapter 1) with a historical perspective, reviewing the ways in which Carl Rogers came to understand the importance of his necessary and sufficient conditions—especially PR. We discuss the current place and importance of this concept and the questions that have arisen about its definition and include several clinical vignettes in which the therapist's PR played a significant role in the process and outcome of the case. We also examine several enduring controversies: whether explicit affirmations on the part of the therapist should be considered legitimate aspects of PR, despite the fact that they violate Rogers's principle of nonjudgmental acceptance; whether there's a true difference between empathy and PR; and whether his three core facilitative attitudes (the therapist's empathy, PR, and genuineness/congruence) are essentially one condition.

In Chapter 2, we turn our attention to the empirical basis of providing PR, summarizing and discussing the studies—most recently, the meta-analyses conducted by our research team—that have investigated the association between PR and therapeutic outcome. The results of these investigations provide the foundation for our contention, elaborated throughout this book, that adopting a broad-based attitude of PR should be the goal of therapists across multiple theoretical traditions. We also consider here the factors that mediate or moderate the association between PR and outcome and note the limitations of many of these studies, specifically the narrow way that PR is operationalized in most assessment measures.

In Chapter 3, we examine the ways in which PR has been modified and reinterpreted by theorists and clinicians within the person-centered community. We examine some of the controversies spurred by these writers, including whether PR can be "faked," whether there are optimal levels of this attitude, and whether a therapist can be both person-centered and eclectic. We note, too, the possibility that the concept itself may now be interpreted differently as a function of the changes in Western culture over the past several decades.

In Chapter 4, we move to discussions of the work of prominent therapists outside the person-centered community who have integrated into their own theoretical systems concepts similar, though not identical, to PR. Among those whom we consider are Marsha Linehan and the concept of "validation," Heinz Kohut and his views about "mirroring," D. W. Winnicott and the "holding environment," John Bowlby and Mary Ainsworth's ideas about a "secure base," and Shari Geller's (and others') concept of "therapeutic presence." The PR-like concepts that this varied group of therapists have proposed suggest that the foundation for greater widespread clinical adoption of PR may already be in place, albeit with terms unassociated with the person-centered community.

Chapter 5 examines the ways in which PR may be expressed in other than psychotherapeutic situations. We first look at the career and message of (Mister)

Fred Rogers, a person who seemed to exemplify the characteristics that Carl Rogers identified as positively regarding. We explore the ways in which the ideologies of these two remarkable men overlap and, again, whether there are implications here for the contemporary practice of psychotherapy. We next summarize the results of our study of the characteristics that graduate students in psychology attribute to the most positively regarding and least positively regarding individual they know. Finalizing our focus on looking at PR in other than clinical settings, the last part of this chapter examines the nature of PR in the burgeoning world of social media. Our belief is that understanding the ways that PR is now understood and experienced by those outside the therapeutic dyad—especially young adults—and the ways that it is manifest in social media can help therapists adopt this attitude in ways that reflect the needs of the next generation of therapy seekers.

In Chapter 6, we strive to identify the specific, active components of PR. We discuss the results of a survey that investigated clients' perceptions of their therapists' most affirming behaviors as well as clients' sense of which of these occurred most frequently during the course of their therapy. We highlight the specific client, therapist, and treatment variables that are significantly associated with client perceptions of the frequency and potency of the PR they've received. We also delve into the results of a qualitative (interview) study that addressed several related topics, including respondents' sense of the effects of their therapists' PR, their beliefs about the consequences of insufficient doses of PR, their ideas about whether therapists could express too much PR, and their sense of what therapists might do to enhance or improve the ways in which they convey this quality. We provide a summary, based on the results of these studies and the case examples in this chapter, of the three constituent factors that we believe underlie PR. Finally, with a nod to the current need for most psychotherapies to be conducted via video conferencing, this chapter analyzes clients' beliefs about the ways in which their therapists' provision of PR has been transformed through teletherapy.

Chapter 7 provides a complement to the previous chapter. That is, in this chapter, we discuss the findings of our research that investigated therapist perceptions of PR. What do a heterogeneous group of therapists consider the most affirming ways of conveying PR? What kinds of PR do they believe they most frequently communicate? How important do they think this attitude is in the overall context of conducting effective psychotherapy? What do they believe PR best accomplishes? Do they imagine that either too much or too little PR can result in therapeutic ruptures? Do they believe there are times when PR has had adverse clinical effects? What factors, including therapeutic orientation and client diagnosis, affect how therapists convey PR to clients?

Although we include numerous illustrations of PR in Chapters 1 through 7, in Chapter 8 we provide examples of the diverse ways in which PR may manifest across long-term therapies. PR is, after all, more of an enduring attitude than it is a discrete act. More specifically, in this chapter, we summarize and discuss the positively regarding ways of four different therapists with four clients: Carl Rogers's therapy with a 20-year-old depressed client; my own work with a woman who suffered from the consequences of severe physical, sexual, and emotional abuse during childhood; the clinical work of Dr. Betsy Glaser, the featured therapist in Terry Wise's 2012 book, *Waking Up: Climbing Through the Darkness*, in treating a grieving, suicidal young woman; and Dr. Amy Wenzel's cognitive behavior therapy (CBT) treatment of a woman dealing with persistent self-deprecating thoughts. These cases reaffirm the variety of ways that PR can be expressed and the need for PR to be modified as a function of the changing needs of different clients as well as therapists' individual styles.

In our last chapter (Chapter 9), we circle back to some of the criticisms leveled at Rogers's ideas about PR, including the idea that this attitude may lead to collusion with a client's defenses or resistance to change; that PR, even in combination with the other facilitative conditions, is likely not sufficient to effectively treat individuals with certain clinical conditions (e.g., borderline personality disorder); that therapist-held attitudes of PR and genuineness are, at times, inevitably at odds; and that traditional ways of providing PR elide the potential positively regarding properties of explicit affirmations, compliments, interpretations, and—even in some cases—confrontations. In summarizing the limitations as well as the considerable benefits of PR as an attitude and set of behaviors, we offer some ideas for how knowledge of PR can be further integrated in mental health training programs across multiple theoretical orientations. We conclude this book by providing recommendations for those therapists who wish to integrate or further their use of PR in their clinical practice. Here we emphasize, more than has typically been noted, the need for therapists to tailor their positively regarding attitudes and behavior to the specific and changing needs of individual clients.

OUR AIMS AND INTENDED AUDIENCE

None of the three coauthors of this book are person-centered therapists. We have studied the works of Carl Rogers, run research labs in which we have guided discussions of his articles and books, and published theoretical pieces and research studies on the topic of PR. We've gone to person-centered conferences and have had extensive discussions with eminent researchers and theorists associated with this community. We've been influenced greatly in our own clinical work by Rogers's ideas—but, again, we have not been immersed in a person-centered community, nor do any of us practice from an exclusively or even primarily person-centered perspective. In these ways, we are perhaps limited in our knowledge. But we believe that there's a certain advantage to our perspective.

The literature on PR has, to date, been written almost entirely by person-centered therapists, and although this is hardly surprising, it is also not ideal. Almost inevitably, there has been a paucity of objective judgment on the validity and generalizability of the concept of PR. We appreciated greatly and learned a great deal from the only other previous book dedicated to PR, one coedited by Jerold Bozarth and Paul Wilkins (2001). Nevertheless, the 16 chapters in that book were all written by person-centered therapists, albeit "from a variety of perspectives within the broad person-centred tradition" (p. viii). Some of the writers in that book were critical of some aspects of Rogers's ideas about PR, and we discuss these views in Chapter 3 of our book, but none of the authors adopted a different perspective—for example, a psychodynamic or CBT perspective—on the clinical worth and place of PR. As writers with a more eclectic stance regarding clinical research and practice, our goal in this book is to offer what we believe is a more balanced, objective, and research-oriented approach to the place of PR in the practice of psychotherapy.

Even as novel therapies emerge, each with its promising initial results and typically overstated convictions, most practitioners across the range of psychotherapeutic approaches now agree that the therapeutic relationship is the key to effective psychotherapy. New approaches to enhancing the relationship, understanding the ways in which it may get derailed and repaired, and explaining the factors that may affect its strength are constantly evolving. The significance of PR in the development and maintenance of the therapeutic relationship is hardly a new idea. Carl Rogers was writing about this over 60 years ago. Now, though, in light of (a) new empirical and conceptual developments in understanding the ways that therapists and clients perceive its most potent and frequently occurring elements, (b) increasing evidence of its significant association to therapeutic outcome, (c) the adoption of PR or variants thereof in a number of contemporary therapies, and (d) the conspicuous absence of PR in multiple spheres of contemporary life, it seems a propitious time to examine the history, evolution, misperceptions, criticisms, and value of PR, with an eye toward arguing for a greater acceptance—albeit within limits—of the role of PR across a wide variety of clients and therapies.

Near the end of his life, Rogers (1986) responded to a question about the future of the person-centered approach to therapy:

> There is only one way in which a person-centered approach can avoid becoming narrow, dogmatic, and restrictive. That is through studies—simultaneously hardheaded and tender-minded—which open new vistas, bring new insights, challenge our hypotheses, enrich our theory, expand our knowledge, and involve us more deeply in an understanding of the phenomenology of human change. (p. 259)

In this regard, our goal is to provide therapists across a variety of theoretical orientations new ways of understanding PR and adopting this stance in clinical practice. Fundamentally, we attempt to provide helpful answers to the following guiding question: How might PR be conceptualized and enacted, post Rogers, in a way that best reflects contemporary needs of clients and contemporary ways of practicing therapy? We hope it will appeal to a wide range of practitioners, including those drawn to humanistic, existential, or spiritual approaches for whom a reconsideration of the role of PR—of listening to and caring deeply for others—will be appealing; those many clinicians who now view the relational elements of their clinical work as foundational; and all therapists looking to increase the effectiveness of their practices.

1

WHAT IS POSITIVE REGARD, AND WHY IS IT IMPORTANT?

What is it worth to be looked at, without judgment, for as long as you need?
—Richard Powers, *The Overstory*

Positive regard (PR) has long been associated with the tenets of Carl Rogers and client-centered (later person-centered) therapy. Put simply, it refers to the therapist's support and acceptance of the client regardless of how the client may behave or present in any given moment. It is not about specific words or behavioral gestures but a consistent attitude—a nonjudgmental and caring attitude, with a touch or more of warmth. Along with the therapist's empathy and genuineness, PR is one of the necessary attitudes for therapeutic change posited by Rogers. PR has historically contained two strands: (a) unconditional positive regard (UPR), essentially acceptance; and (b) positive regard per se, essentially caring and support. This distinction is still maintained within the person-centered approach, but therapists and researchers outside that tradition have typically condensed these two strands into a single, omnibus attitude containing aspects of each. In one form or another, the therapist's provision of PR has become an accepted part of most therapies now practiced.

https://doi.org/10.1037/0000312-002
Understanding and Enhancing Positive Regard in Psychotherapy: Carl Rogers and Beyond, by B. A. Farber, J. Y. Suzuki, and D. Ort

And why not? Everyone wants to be accepted, acknowledged, cared about, and appreciated. Conversely, almost everyone is sensitive to criticism and judgment. William James (1890/1981), the father of American psychology, thought that the need for appreciation was the "deepest principle in human nature" (p. 313). In a contemporary vein, several theorists (e.g., Henriques, 2012; Leary & Allen, 2011) contended that "relational value," the extent to which one feels accepted and valued by important others, is a core human need. Children want to be seen and affirmed, entreating endlessly, "Look at me, Mommy!" Teens and young adults—and many older adults, as well—want their social media messages or pictures "liked" or, even better, commented on or, better still, to "go viral." Athletes want to be "respected" (although this usually means being paid more money). And virtually everyone in a significant relationship wants to feel appreciated and absolutely not taken for granted, ignored, "ghosted," or extensively criticized. We feel more alive, vital, and connected when these needs are met. We feel hurt, isolated, insecure, angry, resentful, invisible, and/or insignificant when we do not feel heard, affirmed, and deeply regarded by important others—or even at times by seemingly non-important others. Many of us are dependent not just on the attention and kindness of loved ones but also, as in Tennessee Williams's (1947) oft-quoted observation, "on the kindness of strangers" (p. 164).

But many questions abound about this general phenomenon. Is being accepted the same as being liked, appreciated, validated, or nonpossessively loved? Are there any downsides to treating individuals in a positively regarding fashion, therapy or otherwise? What are psychotherapy clients' preferred forms for receiving PR—what verbal statements and nonverbal behaviors best serve these needs? What demographic and/or personality factors affect such preferences? Are there cultural differences in the ways in which PR is understood or provided? To what extent is empathy a type of PR? Are there ways for therapists to provide PR to clients that fall outside the definition offered by person-centered psychotherapists? For example, could challenging a client be seen or felt as positively regarding? What types of individuals appear to be immune to these seemingly universal needs? What types of individuals appear to have virtually insatiable needs to be affirmed, appreciated, and loved? What are the immediate and distal effects of being unconditionally accepted and affirmed? What are the immediate and distal effects of not having needs for affirmation fulfilled? Just how healing is receiving PR from others? And what does PR actually heal? Does a steady diet of PR feel superficial—that is, less honest or "deep" or healing than accurate feedback or criticism? Can PR really be provided unconditionally?

These questions seem all the more salient in the current age, one in which politically infused intolerance—exacerbated now (2020–2022) by the great distress caused by the coronavirus pandemic—seems to preclude the ability of many individuals to accept, appreciate, or respect others whose views, gender, religion, sexual orientation, country of origin, immigration status, political affiliation, or ethnicity differ from their own (Schneider, 2013). Hall and Leary (2020) published an article in *Scientific American* contending that Americans are experiencing an "empathy deficit." Annual surveys of the state of civility in America conducted since 2010 have revealed that a substantial majority of Americans believe there is a civility problem in their country. In 2018, fully 93% suggested there was such a problem, with most (69%) identifying it as a major problem (Weber Shandwick, 2018). Arthur C. Brooks (2019), a columnist for *The Washington Post* and occasional op-ed contributor to *The New York Times*, has gone even further, suggesting that in the United States we now live in a "culture of contempt," a phrase that is perhaps the perfect antonym for an attitude of abiding respect and PR for others. He wrote, "The problem in America today is not incivility or intolerance. It's something far worse" (A. C. Brooks, 2019, subhead). Quoting the 19th-century German philosopher Arthur Schopenhauer, he noted that contempt can be understood as "the unsullied conviction of the worthlessness of another" (A. C. Brooks, 2019, para. 5). His partial solution to this crisis is to strive to respond to others' contempt with warmheartedness and humor.

There is something about this proposal that seems at once profound, courageous, and unrealistic. It's a bit like John Lennon's song "Imagine." While there's something wonderful about the notion that we should all be oblivious to religious differences and political borders and thus living life in peace, it's not going to happen. Humans naturally maintain social networks, with strong loyalties to their own "tribe" or social group. More to the point: How many of us could be warmhearted, kind, or smile in response to those who would want to exile, imprison, or harm us or our children for holding views contrary to theirs? A survivor of the horrendous massacre at a mosque in New Zealand in March 2019, someone whose wife was killed in the attack, said the following:

> I lost my wife, but I don't hate the killer. As a person, I love him. . . . I'm sorry I cannot support what he did, but I think somewhere along in his life, maybe he was hurt, but he could not translate that hurt in a positive manner. (*Christchurch Shooting Survivor Says He Forgives His Wife's Killer*, 2019)

Within 2 days of BBC News posting this video to Facebook, there were 1,400 responses, most of which echoed this one person's sentiments:

> Sounds like a good-hearted man, but I do not understand his line of thinking at all if sincere. Regardless of ideology those who would wantonly blow away random non combatants would receive no feeling from me but loathing and contempt.

This, of course, is an extreme situation, one in which finding forgiveness and love would be remarkable. And yet, we sense that Brooks is onto something that Rogers would surely have endorsed—that movement in the general direction of acceptance, of greater numbers of individuals exhibiting an attitude of greater regard for those who are unlike themselves in some significant way, could only be for the good. Another person on this same path is Yale professor Nicholas Christakis. Some may remember that in 2015 he and his wife, also a faculty member at Yale, were pilloried by many Yale students for a remark made by her and seconded by him, suggesting that Yale's edict against culturally insensitive Halloween costumes was an overreaction. They were denounced, taunted, ostracized, and targeted for demonstrations outside their residence by students as well as fellow faculty members. Christakis went out to meet with these protesting students, fully aware of how angry they were. His 2019 book, *Blueprint: The Evolutionary Origins of a Good Society*, advances the argument that the scientific community has overemphasized people's capacity for evil and violence, overlooking our capacity for goodness.

The need for PR inevitably plays out in the setting of the psychotherapist's office. Here especially, clients expect to feel accepted, safe, secure, understood, respected, and appreciated. For some, therapy is the only place—or, at least, the most consistent place—in which they feel so regarded. The therapist's provision of PR, along with other elements that contribute to the creation of an effective therapeutic relationship (e.g., an ability to repair ruptures in the therapeutic alliance), significantly facilitates clients' ability to explore and disclose their most private thoughts and feelings to their therapist (Bozarth, 1996; Farber, 2006; Lietaer, 1984; Suzuki, 2018), their openness to new experience (e.g., Bozarth, 1996), and their capacity to make positive changes in their lives (Farber, Suzuki, & Lynch, 2019; Norcross & Lambert, 2019). Absent these features, clients are unlikely to continue therapy.

A CLINICAL EXAMPLE OF CONSISTENTLY PROVIDED POSITIVE REGARD

Carol is a 35-year-old mother of three children who has been seeing her current therapist for the past 6 months. She had been married for 10 years, was separated for 2 years, and has now been legally divorced from her husband for the past 2 years. She works full-time as a paralegal for a midsize law firm in a large city, a job she thinks is "reasonably good" but that necessitates her children going to an after-school program for several hours each day. She began therapy complaining of having "no time" for herself or friends; feeling "guilty" over her divorce and the children's need to split time between her and her estranged husband; and, most especially, feeling "lonely," "low," and "over-whelmed." Carol denied any suicidal ideation but did acknowledge feeling hopeless at times. She also noted that she had been in therapy before, having sought treatment about 5 years previous when she and her husband began to experience significant marital stress, a situation precipitated by her husband's loss of his job (as a department store manager) and increased alcohol use.

Why, her new therapist wanted to know at the outset of their work together, did Carol decide not to continue seeing her previous therapist? What worked well and not so well in that therapy? What might she be looking for differently in this new treatment? Carol explained,

> My old therapist was OK. She was clearly smart and tried hard to be helpful. She was very professional. She asked good questions and wrote down my answers. We brainstormed ways for me to find more time for myself and I even tried some of them. She had me fill out a form about my mood during the week. She gave me homework assignments, mostly asking me to track when I was feeling down and what was going through my head at the time. But I don't know, I never looked forward that much to going and toward the end I started cancelling some sessions. Something was missing. I think I needed a really strong connection with someone and she just seemed too . . . kind of reminded me of some of the lawyers I work with—competent, reasonably nice people, but too much in their heads. I got your name from my primary care doctor who thought I'd like you. She said you had a "warm presence." I liked that phrase.

Now 6 months into treatment with this new female therapist, Dr. Alexander—someone with a roughly equivalent amount of clinical experience as her first therapist but with a different (more eclectic, primarily humanistic) treatment approach—Carol's depression has remitted only moderately. Nevertheless, she feels more hopeful than she has for a while, believing that she and her therapist have a warm, collaborative relationship and that she is cared about, respected, and understood. She likes, too, that her new therapist shares some-what her own experiences—that Dr. Alexander is also a single mother and can appreciate the difficulties this entails.

What has this new therapist actually done? What is she like as a therapist? And to what extent, if any, has her ability to be positively regarding played a role in this treatment?

Dr. Alexander began her professional career practicing the cognitive behavior therapy (CBT) skills she learned in her doctoral program. She felt competent and helpful but came to increasingly believe that her clients' improvement was based more on her ability to engage and believe in them than in any specific clinical interventions she used. She began reading more about humanistic and relationally oriented psychodynamic therapies and attended several courses and workshops that offered instruction in these areas. She found an experienced person-centered therapist from whom she received weekly supervision and gradually shifted her practice in this direction. She did not entirely eliminate CBT interventions from her clinical repertoire but became more focused on the relationship itself. Consciously, but consonant with the shift in her own professional identity toward person-centered principles, she strove to be consistently genuine (including, at times, self-disclosing), empathic, and positively regarding.

An observer of their sessions would note that Dr. Alexander maintained a positively regarding attitude toward her client. She was consistently nonjudgmental, primarily nodding in response to Carol's difficult disclosures (e.g., that she was rageful and insulting in response to her husband's alcohol use, that she had been "too flirtatious" with a coworker). Often, too, Dr. Alexander was explicitly affirming: for example, noting how hard Carol was working in therapy, how competent she was at her job, and how loving and sensitive she was toward her children. Dr. Alexander's nonverbal behaviors and speech patterns—a softness in her voice and gestures, a ready smile—were also reflective of a caring, supportive attitude. Furthermore, her empathic responses seemed very sensitively attuned to the emotional undertones of Carol's statements—for example, "Seems, then, you really did struggle with holding it together." She appeared friendly and receptive to whatever Carol wanted to discuss. Notably, too, whereas Dr. Alexander was consistently nonjudgmental, she was not as consistently nondirective; that is, she occasionally channeled her CBT background to assess the intensity of Carol's depressive symptoms, including her self-deprecating thoughts.

Whether or not this therapist's approach, one quite discrepant from that of Carol's previous therapist, is what is making her feel more hopeful (though only somewhat less overwhelmed or sad) is impossible to say. A new therapist of any sort, even one with an approach similar to that of her previous therapist, may have elicited comparable, hopeful expectations of progress. Moreover, we cannot parse exactly those ingredients in any therapy that are primarily responsible for therapeutic growth or improvement; multiple variables may contribute to a client's sense that therapy is helpful. Perhaps a psychodynamically oriented therapist would have had as much success with Carol as has Dr. Alexander. Every contemporary therapeutic orientation has practitioners with a wide range of interpersonal skills. But to the extent that the therapeutic alliance has been found to be correlated significantly with therapeutic outcome (Flückiger et al., 2018), the fact that Carol and her new therapist seem to be well attuned and that Carol feels well connected with her is certainly a good sign. And to the extent that PR has also been found to be significantly associated with outcome (Farber, Suzuki, & Lynch, 2019), the fact that this new therapist seems to consistently offer Carol a great deal of acceptance as well as overt support and affirmation suggests that PR may be playing some important role in this therapy.

Furthermore, it may be the case that Carol really is best suited at this point in her life to be working with a therapist who is so positively regarding. We are reminded of a dialogue that Rogers (1951) recounted of a client who had just undergone a second course of psychotherapy (with someone other than Rogers). When asked by this second therapist why this therapy was successful whereas the first was not, the client stated, "You did about the same things he did, but you seemed really interested in me" (p. 60). Whether or not Dr. Alexander's approach, one featuring many humanistic principles, including PR, will ultimately lead to a significant reduction in Carol's depressive symptomatology is unknown—but, again, there does seem to be a good foundation in place.

PR is, at once, an extraordinarily important part of life, a significant aspect of the therapeutic relationship, a well-established factor in therapeutic change, a fundamental aspect of the therapeutic system championed by one of the most influential psychotherapists of the 20th century (Cook et al., 2009), and—surprisingly and somewhat inexplicably—an underresearched and underemphasized construct in the psychotherapy literature. Even as theoretical and empirical work on empathy; therapist genuineness and self-disclosure; and, especially, the therapeutic alliance has remained robust in recent decades, work on PR has been minimal. At least in part, this may be because PR, especially its unconditionality component, has been seen as an imperfect concept—as insufficiently distinguishing between acceptance and approval (e.g., Kensit, 2000) and insufficiently distinguishable from empathy and genuineness (e.g., Wachtel, 2007). Furthermore, whereas published work on these other critical aspects of psychotherapy has been generated by authors representing multiple theoretical systems, the work on PR has, with few exceptions, come from individuals firmly located within the humanistic or specifically person-centered world.

WHAT EXACTLY IS POSITIVE REGARD?

PR is not quite *love* (at least not the romantic kind), nor even *kindness*, though it may contain the caring elements of both. It's a bit closer to *acceptance* or *nonjudgment*, but it also has elements of *respect, liking, affection, validation, warmth, support,* and *affirmation.* Charles Truax, a student of Rogers and later a collaborator, preferred the term "non-possessive warmth" in his own studies of PR (e.g., Truax et al., 1966; Truax & Carkhuff, 1967). PR is not quite unconditional, at least in terms of a client's behavior, but it does veer strongly in that direction. The phrase itself has a somewhat overly intellectualized, academic-sounding feel to it but is, at its heart, so very basic—something we all crave. It's a bit Zen-like in its evenness, though it has more of a connective, interpersonal tissue. It's mostly an attitude but one that includes a strong feeling component and is manifest through all sorts of verbal and nonverbal behaviors.

Thus, PR is a far more complex and far-reaching concept than its critics acknowledge. At times, it has been associated primarily with *acceptance* or a basic *nonjudgmental attitude*; at other times, it has been associated with the therapist's *affirmation* (or *warmth*, *liking*, *prizing*, or *nonpossessive love*) of the client, all of which adds an element of more active movement toward, or caring for, the client. In his dialogue with Martin Buber, Rogers (1961) adopted the phrase "confronting the other," explaining that it meant "accepting the whole potentiality of the other" (p. 55). At times, PR has been coupled with the adjective "unconditional"; at other times, this specifier has been dropped or extensively qualified. For the most part, though, PR has increasingly been thought of primarily in terms of its affirmation/caring dimension rather than the unconditionality component, a trend likely influenced by the editions of *Bergin and Garfield's Handbook of Psychotherapy and Behavior Change* that examined the effects of PR using such terms as "therapist support" and "therapist affirmation" (Orlinsky et al., 1994; Orlinsky & Howard, 1986). This would have surprised and perhaps dismayed Rogers inasmuch as it somewhat redefines his original ideas about PR. But the unconditionality part of PR seems more problematic—is it really possible?—and overt affirmation and/or support and caring strike many as more potent catalysts of behavior change.

Rogers himself offered multiple definitions, sometimes searching for synonyms for an overall state or attitude, sometimes advocating for two different varieties (affirmation/caring, unconditionality) of this attribute—and rarely using the same words to explain this concept in his books, chapters, articles, or filmed interviews. Similarly, those attempting to operationalize this concept by designing measures for it have been inconsistent in regard to whether it is best understood and assessed as a single construct primarily reflecting affirmation/caring or as a dual construct reflecting this affectively laden dimension as well as a dimension reflecting unconditionality of acceptance.

A basic problem here is that acts of affirmation reflective of liking or caring or nonpossessive loving are not the same as an overall attitude of acceptance or nonjudgment. As Mearns (1994) argued, accepting somebody is different from liking them; "liking" is conditional and often based on shared beliefs or values. He believed that client-centered therapists should strive to be "beside" their clients, not "on their side" (p. 54). Similarly, Gelso (2019) contended that therapists should emphasize empathy and eschew "too much direct support" (p. 30). His sense was that PR or affirmation is best conveyed by "the therapist's communication to the patient that the patient has a right to experience what s/he experiences [and] has a right to his or her feelings" (p. 38).

Furthermore, therapists' words or actions that seem to be signs of valuing clients and embracing their being tend to have a different, more positively valenced feeling than words or actions reflective of an accepting, nonjudgmental stance. Telling a client, "I care about you" or "I really value the work you're doing here" is likely to generate a greater affective response and a greater sense of connection to the therapist than "I can understand why you did that" or a straightforward "Hmm hmm." Similarly, smiling at a client will likely elicit a different affective reaction than head-nodding that reflects acceptance. Although it can be argued that over time, unconditional acceptance of another—the total or near-total absence of judgment—has significant beneficial effects on a person's sense of self and ability to thrive, actions reflective of acceptance are arguably less impactful than overt behaviors or words reflecting a sense of warmth, support, and caring. Strict acceptance with no emotional tone can have the veneer of—and can be misunderstood as—a neutral response, leaving some clients frustrated and unsure of what the therapist really thinks of them. That said, one can be nonjudgmental while conveying a sense of warmth—a combination that Rogers seemed to have mastered.

Another issue is this: Should both the affirmation/caring piece and the acceptance/unconditionality piece of PR be viewed as existing on a continuum? Whereas Rogers initially implied that the therapist's acceptance of their client needed to be unequivocal or unqualified, he also pointed out that "unconditionality" may have its limits—that it was unlikely to exist in absolute terms but rather should be seen as an ideal that one should strive toward. Affirmation, too, can be seen as varying, both in terms of the consistency with which it is offered to clients and the extent to which it contains a sense of warmth. On the low end of a hypothetical warmth continuum, affirmation can be only mildly warm; on the high end, it can be suffused with a great deal of overt caring and even, in Rogers's terms, "non-possessive love."

Further complicating the issue of definition, many theorists, including Rogers, have written about PR in ways that clearly include empathy as part of its description. Here is Rogers (1961), in *On Becoming a Person: A Therapist's View of Psychotherapy*, describing what he feels is most important in accepting another:

> I have found it of enormous value when I can permit myself to understand the other person. The way in which I have worded this statement may seem strange to you. Is it necessary to permit oneself to understand another? I think it is. Our first reaction to most of the statements (which we hear from other people) is an evaluation or judgment, rather than an understanding of it. When someone

expresses some feeling, attitude or belief, our tendency is almost immediately to feel "that's right," or "that's stupid," "that's abnormal," "that's unreasonable," "that's incorrect," "that's not nice." Very rarely do we permit ourselves to understand precisely what the meaning of the statement is to the other person. (p. 16)

In fact, this quote implies strongly that empathy and understanding are far more critical to a stance of PR than is affirmation—at least, forms of affirmation that suggest judgment, even positively tinged judgment.

Operationally, on a manifest level, there is little to distinguish between empathy and PR (Wilkins, 2000/2001). Studies have consistently found a high degree of overlap between these two concepts (e.g., Barrett-Lennard, 2015; Elliott et al., 2019; Gurman, 1977; Suzuki & Farber, 2016; Truax & Carkhuff, 1967; Watson & Geller, 2005). Measures of PR contain items that tap empathy (e.g., Truax & Carkhuff, 1967), and the converse is true, as well (e.g., Burns & Nolen-Hoeksema, 1992; Watson, 1999). According to many theorists within the client-centered tradition (e.g., Bozarth, 2001; Brodley & Schneider, 2001), PR is conveyed primarily through the therapist's empathy. "Empathy," wrote Bozarth (1996), "is the 'vessel' by which the therapist communicates unconditional positive regard in the most pure way" (p. 55). In fact, from this perspective, the curative power of empathy is due to its positively regarding element. Furthermore, much like PR itself, empathy can be conveyed in multiple ways (Bohart & Greenberg, 1997; Elliott et al., 2019). Empathic responsiveness on the part of therapists is certainly not restricted to the therapist's checking his or her understanding of the client's communication.

We're left with the question, then, as to whether empathy and PR are distinct qualities or whether they inevitably and extensively overlap. It is hard to imagine a scenario in which the therapist's empathy does not also feel positively regarding to a client. A therapist who tries their best to understand the client's experiential world—"It feels to me that you're really struggling with these feelings, this seems so very hard for you"—is showing the client that they are important, deserving to be understood deeply and taken seriously. Nevertheless, there are those who believe there are significant conceptual differences between these concepts. Gelso (2019), for example, stated emphatically that "empathy should not be conflated with caring or positive regard" (p. 33). His sense here is that therapists can empathize with clients without especially caring for them. Our sense is somewhat different. We believe that one can be positively regarding without being empathic but that, as above, true empathy nearly inevitably reflects an affirming attitude—a sense of "I care enough about you to attempt to find out what you're truly experiencing."

Some authors have also contended that it is the therapist's *congruence*, also known as *genuineness*, that is invariably confounded with his or her communication of PR. Lietaer (1984) believed that these qualities are complementary—

that is, two sides of the same "openness" coin. In his formulation, genuineness represents an openness toward self and PR an openness toward others: "The more I accept myself and am able to be present in a comfortable way with everything that bubbles up in me, without fear or defense, the more I can be receptive to everything that lives in my client" (p. 44).

Finally, several person-centered authors have suggested that Rogers's three core attitudes should really be considered a single concept with multiple strands (e.g., Mearns & Cooper, 2005; Mearns & Thorne, 2000; Wilkins, 2000/2001). Bozarth (1998), for example, suggested that the three conditions are inherently linked, "ultimately and functionally, one condition" (p. 80). According to his model, congruence (or genuineness or authenticity) can be thought of as a state of readiness within the therapist that allows them to experience the client through empathic understanding; in turn, empathic understanding is the way the therapist conveys UPR. The penultimate assumption is that UPR is the curative factor in person-centered therapy. Why "penultimate"? Because, according to Bozarth (1998), the therapist's UPR is, in fact, a mediating variable: UPR works because it leads to the activation or enhancement of clients' natural tendency toward growth (i.e., their "actualizing tendency").

> It is the [actualizing] tendency that is the fundamental curative factor lying within the person. The reference to unconditional positive regard as the curative factor assumes the thwarting of the natural tendency; hence, making it necessary that the client become more directly connected with the actualizing tendency through unconditional positive regard. (p. 82)

Yet another way of attempting to define PR is by describing what it is not—or, rather, offering a case illustration wherein it has been lacking. Here, Rogers (1986) suggested that whereas he was, for the most part, accepting of his client, in one crucial exchange he failed to provide PR in accord with his beliefs and principles:

> I show real acceptance of her [my client's] desire to be dependent, to rely on me as the authority who will give the answers. Notice that I accept her *wish* to be dependent. This does *not* mean that I will behave in such a way as to meet her expectations. I can more easily accept her dependent feelings, because I know where I stand, and I know that I will not be her authority figure, even though I am perceived as such.
>
> But at one point my acceptance is not complete. She says, in effect, "I'll talk more to help you in your task," and instead of completely accepting her perception of the relationship, I make two futile attempts to change her perception. I respond, in effect, "What we are doing is to help you, not me." She disregards this, and no damage is done to the process. (p. 150)

In reading through the transcript of this interview, it's difficult to delineate any specific examples of Rogers's acceptance of this client. That is, there are no specific words Rogers uses that explicitly indicate he accepts his client unconditionally; neither does he offer any explicit words of validation, liking, or caring. Rather, for the most part, his empathy—his reflection of her feelings or thoughts without judgment—is what constitutes acceptance within this session. To some extent, too, there's a bit of humor, some banter and laughter between them that suggests a degree of warmth. Rogers's perceived lapse is when he attempts to correct this client's perception of why she is disclosing to him. She says, "So the more I talk, the more I'm helping you to get through to me, is that right?" A few conversational turns later he says, "And one other thing that you said: that you're trying to help *me*. I guess I hope that what we're doing here will help *you*" (Rogers, 1986, p. 145).

In fact, despite her awkward phrasing, she's not wrong: Her disclosures in therapy do allow Rogers to be helpful to her. While her disclosures are not, strictly speaking, for Rogers's sake—as he takes pains to point out—they do provide the material for him to do the work and allow him to know her better. He's being somewhat pedantic, an unusual stance for him. But more basically, it is his attempt to correct her, to not accept her version of the truth even as it is at odds with his version of the basic truth of therapy, that is antithetical to his mandate for the therapist to be unconditionally accepting. To borrow from the parlance of improvisational theater, positively regarding therapists aim to respond to clients with "Yes, and . . ." and aspire to eliminate the impulse toward "No, but . . ." from their repertoire.

POSITIVE REGARD VERSUS UNCONDITIONAL POSITIVE REGARD

The use of the terms *positive regard* and *unconditional positive regard* has led to a fair amount of confusion. At times, these terms have been used as synonyms; at other times, researchers and clinicians have attempted to distinguish between the two. In his 1957 paper, Rogers used the term *unconditional positive regard* and identified two distinctive components: *unconditionality* (essentially acceptance) and *regard* (essentially warmth or liking). In his 1959 paper, he used the terms *positive regard* and *unconditional positive regard*.

Initial efforts to measure Rogers's facilitative conditions attempted to distinguish between these two concepts. The most commonly used measure of Rogers's facilitative conditions, the Barrett-Lennard Relationship Inventory (BLRI; Barrett-Lennard, 1962, 1986), utilized two subscales: Level of Regard, "the overall level or tendency of one person's affective response to another" (Barrett-Lennard, 1986, p. 440); and Unconditionality of Regard, the extent to which "regard . . . is stable" (p. 443). However, subsequent research indicated that the Unconditionality of Regard subscale was less reliable and valid than the other three subscales of the BLRI (Barrett-Lennard, 1962; Cramer, 1986). As a result, the Unconditionality of Regard subscale has typically been excluded in studies using the BLRI scales. In addition, as alluded to earlier, the mainstream clinical literature has tended to focus more on the "positive regard" strand of Rogers's concept than the "unconditionality" strand—in part because many have found "unconditionality" an untenable clinical idea. For these reasons, following this chapter, we almost exclusively use the term *positive regard* to refer to the overall concept that Rogers had in mind.

CARL ROGERS, POSITIVE REGARD, AND THE DEVELOPMENT AND ASSUMPTIONS OF CLIENT-CENTERED THERAPY

Where does PR fit in terms of the origins and development of client-centered therapy? Early in his career, in his 1942 book, *Counseling and Psychotherapy: Newer Concepts in Practice*, Rogers alluded to the importance of the therapist's provision of PR, although he never used this term. He noted four qualities he considered essential for a helpful therapeutic relationship, the first of which he described as "warmth and responsiveness on the part of the counselor which makes rapport possible" (p. 87). This quality, he suggested, "expresses itself in a genuine interest in the client and an acceptance of him as a person" (p. 87). The second quality that Rogers described in this book is somewhat similar, marked by the use again of the word "acceptance": "By the counselor's acceptance of his statements, by the understanding attitude which pervades the counseling interview, the client comes to recognize that all feelings and attitudes may be expressed" (p. 88). To complete this list: The third quality noted was the need for therapeutic "limits" (i.e., boundaries), in terms, for example, of the length of time of sessions; and the fourth quality was the need for the therapist (or "counselor," in Rogers's words) to be clear that sessions needed to stay focused on the client's needs. According to Rogers (1942),

> the skillful therapist refrains from intruding his own wishes, his own reactions or biases, into the therapeutic situations . . . advice, suggestions, pressure to follow one course of action rather than another—these are out of place in therapy. (p. 89)

Subsequently, Rogers would combine these first two elements into his notion of PR—though again, throughout his career, he wavered as to whether these were really one overall attitude or two overlapping attitudes (affirmation/caring and nonjudgmental acceptance).

What is also intriguing is that in this book, Rogers (1942) strongly refuted the practice of offering reassurance and encouragement to clients. The use of phrases such as "you're doing well" or "you're improving," contended Rogers, "denies the problem which exists . . . denies the feeling that the individual has about the problem [such that the individual] does not feel free to bring his less acceptable impulses to the clinical situation" (p. 21). Furthermore, he noted, the client should expect "neither blame nor oversympathetic indulgence and praise . . . [nor] undue support nor unwelcome antagonism" (p. 90). And here is a crucial reminder of what Rogers did not mean when he wrote about his way of doing therapy: "Therapy, it cannot be stressed enough, is not merely being 'nice' to a person in trouble" (p. 105). Despite this clearly stated sentence, critics of Rogers have assumed that this is exactly and entirely what his therapeutic approach is about. Furthermore, as we see later (Chapter 6), clients themselves believe that overtly sympathetic and complimentary statements of their therapist are valid forms of PR.

Carl Rogers's Early Life Experiences

If we back up a step, we can examine some of the sources that influenced Rogers's approach, including his insistence on fully accepting the person of the client. A good starting point would be his own history, including the values of the household in which he grew up. Much of the material that follows comes from Rogers (1980) himself, as well as from Kirschenbaum's (2007) comprehensive biography of Rogers.

Born in 1902 in the suburbs of Chicago, Carl was raised in an insular, religious community that eschewed secular influences—"the place where the saloons end and the churches begin" was the town's slogan—and in line with this sentiment, the community enacted legislation to protect residents from uncensored movies, games (e.g., gambling), and alcohol consumption, even limiting access to information on contraception and STDs.

This ideology, which was prevalent in Rogers's home environment as well, restricted severely his social life. As fundamentalist Protestant Christians, Carl's parents believed that as God's chosen people, it was somewhat unfitting for their children to socialize with "those who were not so favored" (Kirschenbaum, 2007, p. 6)—in other words, less religious individuals. Reflecting on his parents' views, Carl said,

> I think the attitude toward persons outside our family can be summed up in this way: other persons behave in dubious ways which we do not approve of in our family. . . . Other people go play cards, go to movies, smoke, dance, drink, and engage in other activities, some unmentionable. (Rogers, 1980, p. 28)

Carl's sense of isolation was deeply connected with an overall ethos of judgment of others and by separateness from others. Even when Carl had opportunities to interact with his peers, he struggled to feel accepted socially.

Despite earning a reputation for being exceptionally bright—he read by age 4—Carl's sensitive nature and frail build made him easy prey for teasing and bullying. Moreover, his tearful reactions to being teased and his unwillingness to respond in kind led to his being described as "thin-skinned" and perpetuated the teasing. As Carl grew older, the teasing and bullying lessened, but his loneliness did not. When he was 13, his parents moved to a farm in a remote area in Illinois, largely as a way to protect Carl and his siblings from "the corrupting influences of city and suburbs" (Kirschenbaum, 2007, p. 9). In Carl's case, their efforts were, perhaps, too successful. Carl spent his high school years focusing exclusively on school and the farm. Not only did he avoid all social activities outside his home, but he also never brought any friends to visit the family's 300-acre farm.

As an escape from his loneliness and social distress, Carl turned to books, and he frequently spent hours alone engrossed in fantasy and adventure stories. "I get pretty lonesome," Carl wrote in his diary, "but I have a fine time with my new books" (Kirschenbaum, 2007, p. 16). Although being an avid reader provided comfort, his parents disapproved, preferring that he use his time on more practical chores. To this end, Carl recalls his mother's frequent complaint: "There you go again with your nose in a book" (Kirschenbaum, 2007, p. 4).

Whereas Carl's parents clearly loved and cared for their children, attended to their spiritual and practical needs, and fostered their strong work ethic and entrepreneurial spirit, there is no documentation of Carl ever writing or saying anything about his relationship with his parents that conveys warmth, intimacy, or unconditional acceptance. Their strict discipline and unbending expectations for religious adherence were not balanced with acceptance and positive regard, creating little space for Carl to develop an appreciation for his own values, talents, and uniqueness. In fact, it wasn't until high school that Carl experienced some much-needed acceptance from a teacher who taught him, in Carl's own words, "that it was alright to be original and unique" (Kirschenbaum, 2007, p. 15).

That this was the lived experience of a founding father of humanistic psychotherapy might, at first glance, seem surprising. Where did Carl Rogers learn the power of connection and warmth? How did he come to so deeply appreciate the need for acceptance? Having had an extremely prescribed experience as a child, how did he become aware of the potency of nondirective support? Arguably, what the first 2 decades of Carl's life taught him above all was the detrimental effects of insufficient nurturing conditions. The love and practical support provided by Carl's parents did not sufficiently nurture his emotional needs nor foster his individuality. Growing up in an environment in which he felt that acceptance was conditional left him feeling inadequate and lonely. Experiencing new, more supportive and accepting environments empowered Carl to live more congruently, including marrying a woman against his parents' wishes and switching careers from ministry to psychology. Moreover, these early experiences provided the foundation for his search for a method of healing that would provide exactly what he so missed.

Professional Influences

What about his professional influences? As many have noted, but none so incisively as Kramer (1995), one of the great influences on Rogers's theories and psychotherapy model was Otto Rank. Originally a member of Freud's inner circle and arguably the most original thinker among this group, Rank was exiled when he disputed the primacy of the father and of the Oedipus complex in human development and the origins of neurosis. Rank (1936/1978) wrote extensively about creativity and individuation, focusing on the notion of self-development. Neurosis, according to Rank, arises as a result of the failure to develop one's potential—to assert and affirm oneself fully as an individual. Among many others, Ernest Becker (1973) was greatly drawn to Rank's ideas and incorporated many of them in his Pulitzer Prize-winning book, *The Denial of Death*.

Rank believed that individuals experience two lifelong and paradoxical fears: the fear of merger (with the anticipated loss of one's individuality and uniqueness) and the fear of separation (with the anticipated loss of one's connection to others and all of nature). A partial solution to this, he thought, was through connection to another who accepts both one's uniqueness and difference. Human suffering, contended Rank, could only be alleviated by another who "accepts us as we are" (cited in Kramer, 1995, p. 72). Accordingly, a therapist should not assume the role of an authority figure who maintains a posture, per psychoanalytic dicta, of strict neutrality, anonymity, and abstinence but rather of an assistant ego (Rank, 1936/1978, p. 68), someone with whom the patient can bond in order to ultimately find their own way.

Significantly, and clearly foreshadowing Rogers, Rank believed it was the relationship per se, not the therapist's insights, that was healing. As Kramer (1995) explained, Rank believed that "healing, or making whole, comes from mutual recognition not intellectual understanding" (p. 74). What the client needed from the therapist, thought Rank (1936/1978), was an emotional experience with a therapist in the "here and now" (p. 39). And the specific emotional experience he named was love: "In love and through love the individual can accept himself, his own will, because the other does, an other does" (p. 64). The therapist best accomplishes this—demonstrates love—through empathic understanding of his or her client, a merger of one ego with another. Or, as Rank poetically explained, "The ego needs a Thou in order to become a Self" (p. 290).

Here we are in the realm of the philosopher Martin Buber (1937), whose ideas about "I–Thou" relationships influenced both Rank and Rogers. I–Thou relationships, in contrast to "I–It" relationships, are those in which the other is not separated by discrete bounds. Rather, these relationships are marked by merger and connection; the relationship itself is the dominant mode of perception. According to Buber, all real living is meeting. I–Thou encounters involve the whole being of each person, a revocation of the boundaries between two individuals in the service of true communion. While heretical at the time, all these overlapping concepts proposed to account for therapeutic healing—mutual recognition, empathic understanding, merger and connection, the primacy of the relationship—are now standard fare in most forms of psychotherapy, especially contemporary relational psychodynamic therapy (Wachtel, 2008).

Rogers acknowledged explicitly that he was influenced by Rank's ideas. In fact, he noted that he became "infected with Rankian ideas" (Kirschenbaum, 1979, p. 95), specifically in regard to individuals' capacity for being self-directed, the need for therapy to be relationally oriented, and the clinical importance of staying in the here and now. Notably, too, Rogers came to appreciate the need for a therapist's *empathic understanding*, a term employed by Rank well before Rogers used this phrase in his 1951 book, *Client-Centered Therapy: Its Current Practice, Implications, and Theory*. The primary intermediary between Rank and Rogers was Jessie Taft, a social worker and patient (and then friend and biographer) of Rank's who was extremely taken by Rank's ideas. Taft's presentations of Rank's theories about psychotherapy to the Society for the Prevention of Cruelty to Children in Rochester, where Rogers was working (as director of the Child Study Department), was instrumental in Rogers becoming familiar and enamored with Rankian ideas about how psychotherapy should be conducted.

Kramer (1995) also elucidated the fundamental overlap between PR and empathy. "Empathic understanding," noted Kramer,

> is a form of nonpossessive love that the ancient Greeks called *Agape*—to distinguish it from *Eros*, a grasping possessive love that insists on its own desires being met. . . . Rogers defined Agape as a listening to oneself, as well as a listening love for the other individual. (p. 88)

Thus, both empathy and PR contain this element of nonpossessive love—a sense of understanding, accepting, and caring for the client as a separate person.

Rogers continued to hone his appreciation for individuals' potential for growth through a healing relationship. The epigraph to *Client-Centered Therapy: Its Current Practice, Implications, and Theory* was taken from Ralph Waldo Emerson's 1838 speech to the graduating class of Harvard Divinity School:

> We mark with light in the memory the few interviews we have had, in the dreary years of routine and of sin, with souls that made our souls wiser; that spoke what we thought; that told us what we knew; that gave us leave to be what we inly were. (Rogers, 1951, epigraph)

It is easy to see how these words would exemplify what Rogers had in mind for his new form of psychotherapy—a relationship or experience in which clients were accepted such that they became what they were "inly" meant to be. "This book," noted Rogers (1951) in the preface,

> is about a client in my office who sits there by the corner of the desk, struggling to be himself, yet deathly afraid of being himself—striving to see his experience as it is, wanting to *be* that experience, and yet deeply fearful of the prospect. (p. x)

In the opening pages of this book, Rogers (1951) turned quickly to delineating the basic helping stance of the therapist. Here, a bit of irony in that he implicitly disparaged those therapists (i.e., psychoanalysts) who do not believe that respect for others is fundamental:

> Do we tend to treat individuals as persons of worth, or do we subtly devalue them by our attitudes and behavior? Is our philosophy one in which respect for the individual is uppermost? . . . Among psychologists and psychiatrists there are those with similar views but there are also many whose concept of the individual is that of an object to be dissected, diagnosed, manipulated. (pp. 20–21)

Those who choose to practice client-centered therapy, he contended, are those who already have a "deep respect for the significance and worth of each person" (Rogers, 1951, p. 21), often because they have a deep sense of self-respect. And how, according to Rogers, should a therapist implement this attitude of respect and regard for others in doing the work of therapy? While eschewing any specific words, phrases, or nonverbal behavior, Rogers suggested that one avenue with which to demonstrate PR is through empathy, an intense effort to understand and thus validate another:

> The counselor says in effect, "To be of assistance to you, I will put aside myself—the self of ordinary interaction—and enter into your world of perception as completely as I am able. I will become, in a sense another self for you—an alter ego of your own attitudes and feelings—a safe opportunity for you to discern yourself more clearly, to experience yourself more truly and deeply, to choose more significantly" . . . to focus my whole attention and effort upon understanding and perceiving as the client perceives and understands, is a striking operational demonstration of the belief I have in the worth and the significance of this individual client. (Rogers, 1951, p. 35)

In this passage, we also hear clear reflections of Rank's influence. Rogers, much like Rank, employed the notion of an *alter ego*, someone both outside of and in communion with the client in the service of reflecting the client's worth back to themselves. In considering what made a difference to one client in client-centered therapy, Rogers contended that it was essentially a sense of acceptance: "It was only when another self looked upon her behavior without shame or emotion that she could look upon it in the same way" (Rogers, 1951, p. 40). He reminded readers, too, that his idea of acceptance was essentially one of nondirectiveness; acceptance, as he meant it, does not include overt support or praise for any decision or action. It is support only in the sense that the therapist is supportive (i.e., consistently accepting) of the client.

> It appears that in the client's experience, particularly if the problems have been deep-seated, the only stable portion of experience is the unfailing hour of acceptance by the therapist. In this sense client-centered therapy is experienced as supporting, as an island of constancy in a sea of chaotic difficulty, though it is not "supportive" or approving in the superficial sense. (Rogers, 1951, p. 71)

"Acceptance" and "respect for the individual" are terms used throughout this 1951 volume (including the index). Notably, "positive regard," a term with more of a sense of overt affirmation and caring, is never mentioned.

Rogers credits his student at the University of Chicago, Stanley Standal, with introducing the term "positive regard" to the lexicon of client-centered therapy in his 1954 PhD thesis ("The Need for Positive Regard: A Contribution to Client-Centered Theory"). Standal, by the way, had a rather rocky subsequent career. He founded a therapeutic community in Utah based on humanistic principles of growth and change and was apparently a charismatic but quite damaged leader who suffered from alcoholism, was married five times, was indicted on charges of statutory rape (of one of his followers), and fled the country. The consensus among those who posted thoughts following his 2008 death was that he was a sensitive, passionate, poetic soul, full of vitality—but also a dysfunctional and tormented man, someone whom you either passionately loved or hated.

THE 1957 PAPER: THE NECESSARY AND SUFFICIENT CONDITIONS OF THERAPEUTIC PERSONALITY CHANGE

Carl Rogers began practicing psychology in 1928; he died in 1987. Thus, it was exactly the midpoint of his career (1957) when he published his paper on the necessary and sufficient conditions of therapeutic change. This paper is arguably the most successful of his many attempts to clarify and render testable the ideas behind client-centered therapy that he articulated originally in 1942 in *Counseling and Psychotherapy: Newer Concepts in Practice.*

As he would be at other points in his career, Rogers was frustrated by the lackluster response to these well-formulated ideas by those outside his own circle of influence (Farber et al., 1996; Kirschenbaum & Henderson, 1989). Nevertheless, in retrospect, this paper might be considered the true beginning of the age of relational psychotherapy: "The publication of this classic article seems to have catalyzed a shift in the way that many thought about the putative mechanisms of psychotherapeutic change" (Farber & Lane, 2002, p. 175). The shift was from (a) assuming that technical expertise on the part of therapists, especially in terms of choice and timing of interventions, was essential to therapeutic success to (b) the idea that the relationship per se was critical.

Rogers greatly approved of Standal's term "positive regard" and adopted it in this paper. He cited it as one of the necessary and sufficient conditions for therapeutic change, describing it as follows:

> To the extent that the therapist finds himself experiencing a warm acceptance of each aspect of the client's experience as being a part of that client, he is experiencing unconditional positive regard. This . . . means that there are no conditions of acceptance, no feeling of "I like you only if you are thus and so." It means a "prizing" of the person, as Dewey has used that term. It is at the opposite pole from a selective evaluating attitude—"You are bad in these ways, good in those." It involves as much feeling of acceptance for the client's expression of negative, "bad," painful, fearful, defensive, abnormal feelings as for his expression of "good," positive, mature, confident, social feelings, as much acceptance of ways in which he is inconsistent as of ways in which he is consistent. It means a caring for the client, but not in a possessive way or in such a way as simply to satisfy the therapist's own needs. It means a caring for the client as a separate person, with permission to have his own feelings, his own experiences. (Rogers, 1957, p. 98)

The Dewey reference here is to John Dewey, the American philosopher ("pragmatism"), psychologist, and advocate for progressive education. In Dewey's (1939) terms, *prizing* (appreciating something) is to be distinguished from *appraising* (assigning a value to something). Caring parents, suggested Dewey, do not assign rankings to their children. Thus, Rogers's conceptualization of UPR here blends two components, caring and acceptance/unconditionality: The therapist has a warm and positive response to the client regardless of what experiences or attitudes the client may bring to bear in therapy. But, as in his earlier writings, Rogers appears to emphasize more heavily the acceptance/unconditionality component than the warmth or caring component, as indicated by representative statements in a hypothetical Q-sort task (an assessment tool) he proposed in this same paper to characterize the therapeutic relationship: "I feel no revulsion at anything the client says," "I feel neither approval nor disapproval of the client and his statements—simply acceptance," "I feel warmly toward the client—toward his weaknesses and problems as well as his potentialities," "I am not inclined to pass judgment on what the client tells me," and "I like the client" (1957, p. 98).

Of these five items, only one ("I feel warmly toward the client—toward his weaknesses and problems as well as his potentialities") integrates unconditionality with warmth, while three items focus exclusively on unconditionality, and only one item ("I like the client") emphasizes warmth alone. Rogers added, as a footnote, that "completely unconditional positive regard would never exist except in theory" but that therapists may experience the unconditional specifier toward their clients in certain moments, while at other times experiencing "only a conditional positive regard—and perhaps at times a negative regard, though this is not likely in effective therapy" (Rogers, 1957, p. 98). We see, then, a bit of a paradox here: that even as he adopted the term "unconditional positive regard" and emphasized this attitude more than expressions of warmth or caring, Rogers "fudged" a bit, allowing that a constant, unmodified "unconditional" attitude on the part of a therapist is not actually possible.

An often-overlooked part of this paper is that Rogers actually specified six conditions for change, not just the three (the therapist's congruence or genuineness, empathy, and PR) typically delineated. These other three conditions included the need for two persons to be in "psychological contact" (i.e., in a relationship); for the client to be in "state of incongruence, being vulnerable or anxious" (i.e., that there is a discrepancy between felt experience and self-image); and, most germane to this discussion, that the therapist's communication, to the client, of empathy and PR "is to a minimal degree achieved" (Rogers, 1957, p. 96). What the therapist believes they are achieving in terms of providing empathy and PR is irrelevant if the client does not experience these qualities to at least a minimal extent. Rogers contended, too, in this paper that clinical "techniques" in various therapies—including interpretations, dream analysis, and "reflection of feelings"—are neither necessary nor sufficient; rather, according to his clinical model, they are useful only insofar as they permit the therapist to convey the core attitudes of genuineness, empathy, and PR. Whereas "an interpretation may be given in a way which communicates the unconditional positive regard of the therapist . . . interpretations may [also] be rendered in a way which indicates the highly conditional regard of the therapist" (p. 103). Being smart is not nearly as important or helpful as maintaining a consistently accepting attitude toward one's client.

THE 1959 PAPER: A THEORY OF THERAPY, PERSONALITY, AND INTERPERSONAL RELATIONSHIPS, AS DEVELOPED IN THE CLIENT-CENTERED FRAMEWORK

In a more fully developed treatise on client-centered theory, Rogers (1959) again expressed his appreciation to Rank, particularly the ways in which the latter crystallized Rogers's sense that the connection with the client was paramount, a better way of conducting therapy than imposing one's views or expertise on the client's experience (p. 187). Rogers also used this invited chapter (within an edited book) to elaborate on each of the components of his theory, noting that his formulations here were based primarily on his clinical work: "For a period now approaching thirty years, I have spent probably an average of 15 to 20 hr [*sic*] per week, except during vacation periods, in endeavoring to understand and be of therapeutic help to these individuals" (p. 188). At the low end, then—assuming he worked 45 weeks a year and had 15 clinical hours a week for 30 years—Rogers had already accumulated over 20,000 therapy hours. Among his other observations about this clinical experience was his firm belief that "man lives essentially in his own personal and subjective world, and even his most objective functioning, in science, mathematics, and the like, is the result of subjective purpose and subjective choice" (p. 191). Out of this and several other convictions—for example, that people are inherently directed toward growth (that is, have an actualizing tendency)—he came to his belief that the therapist needs to strive to experience, understand, and accept deeply individuals' subjective worlds.

Much of the lengthy (73-page) chapter by Rogers is dedicated to providing working definitions of the terms he uses in his theories of human development and therapeutic work (e.g., actualizing tendency, self-experience, openness to experience, psychological adjustment, conditions of worth). As part of this effort, he offered definitions of PR as well as UPR. He described PR as follows:

> If the perception by me of some self-experience in another makes a positive difference in my experiential field, then I am experiencing positive regard for that individual. In general, positive regard is defined as including such attitudes as warmth, liking, respect, sympathy, acceptance. (Rogers, 1959, p. 208)

Here, Rogers proffers some commonly used terms (e.g., warmth, liking) that are encompassed by the broader construct of PR. But note, too, that this definition includes the word "sympathy," an unusual word for Rogers and one many would probably swap out for "compassion." But we suspect that

Rogers is referring primarily to empathy in his use of this word. Notably, too, he includes "acceptance" as part of this definition—a term that, in the past, he usually reserved for UPR.

Rogers's definition of unconditional positive regard (following) seems somewhat dense and cumbersome; typically, he wrote in a more lucid, user-friendly fashion. But in a book with the title *Psychology: A Study of a Science* and with chapters from many other notable psychologists of the time (e.g., Henry Murray, David Rapaport, Raymond Cattell, Solomon Asch, Talcott Parsons), he likely wanted to define his theoretical concepts carefully, comprehensively, and as scientifically as possible.

> If the self-experiences of another are perceived by me in such a way that no self-experience can be discriminated as more or less worthy of positive regard than any other, then I am experiencing unconditional positive regard for this individual. To perceive oneself as receiving unconditional regard is to perceive that of one's self-experiences none can be discriminated by the other individual as more or less worthy of positive regard. Putting this in simpler terms, to feel unconditional positive regard towards another is to "prize" him. . . . This means to value the person, irrespective of the differential values which one might place on his specific behaviors. (Rogers, 1959, p. 208)

In this description, Rogers attempted to simplify this concept by offering a single synonym ("prizing") for UPR. However, prizing, as the word is commonly used and as Dewey meant it, has more of a sense of validation and affirmation than acceptance. Rogers's attempts here to discriminate between these two types of PR are only minimally successful in our view. Moreover, as we noted earlier in this chapter, most researchers and clinicians outside the person-centered tradition now refer to a single PR concept, one that is closer in meaning to Rogers's first definition here than that of his description of UPR.

Rogers argued that therapy is often necessary because many individuals suffer from *conditions of worth* that have been laid down early in their lives, a sense that they can be cared about, fully accepted, and loved only if they act, think, and behave in prescribed ways. That is, the message internalized—mostly from parents, but also from other family members, teachers, religious leaders, and other significant figures in a community—is that they are only valuable and lovable if they deny or severely restrict significant aspects of who they are and what they feel and believe. Thus, early conditions of worth lessen individuals' ability to experience and accept their true and authentic selves. An example: In her book analyzing Charles Dickens and his works, psychiatrist Gwen Watkins (1987) suggested that Dickens's stories all reflect the fact that he never received what every child needs: "that *what he is*, his self, is valuable and worthy of respect, and that he is loved because this self is lovable" (pp. 22–23).

The goal, then, per Rogers, is to help clients become more congruent and less restrictive in their lives, such that their expressed feelings, behaviors, and beliefs are more consonant with the true nature and full range of their internal experiences. Rogers (1959) believed that to the extent that conditions of worth were experienced in childhood and that the need for UPR (i.e., true acceptance) was not sufficiently met, individuals would have to experience this in other contexts, such as the therapeutic relationship, before they could fully believe that they were worthy of self-love and love from others. Rogers highlighted the potency of this attitude in the therapeutic relationship in effecting change: "Gradually the client can feel more acceptance of all of his own experiences, and this makes him again more of a whole or congruent person, able to function effectively" (Rogers, 1959, p. 208). Or, in the words of Jerold Bozarth (2001), among the most ardent and thoughtful of client-centered theorists, "the client is helped by the freedom from threat, every exposed aspect of self is accepted equally by the therapist" (p. 10).

A notable historical point: In his often-viewed filmed interview with a volunteer client, Gloria (Shostrom, 1965), Rogers was given an opportunity both before and after his 30-minute therapy session to explain the nature of his work. In the preinterview part, he introduced his tripartite model of therapeutic change, used the word "prizing" multiple times, and also spoke of "caring," "acceptance," and "nonpossessive love." Never, though, did he invoke either the phrase "positive regard" or "unconditional positive regard"; neither did he do so in his postinterview review of the therapy he had just conducted. However, in one of his last published pieces, in reviewing his three core conditions, Rogers (1986) reverted to the phrase "unconditional positive regard," suggesting that this attitude consisted of the therapist's acceptance, caring, or prizing. Acceptance, to Rogers, was always key, even as he and others (see Chapters 2 and 3, this volume) occasionally expanded their ideas about the ways in which this quality—and, even more so, affirmation—could be expressed.

PR is hard to define, especially given that Rogers himself couldn't quite settle on its description or whether it consists of one basic phenomenon or two. It's hard to operationalize, as Rogers primarily described an attitude rather than a set or domain of behaviors. It's hard to assess, because it seems to be confounded with other relational attitudes, especially that of empathy. Moreover, even as most therapists across most therapeutic approaches seem to accept the need for treating their clients in a positively regarding fashion, few outside the humanistic tradition use this phrase to describe this practice.

Nevertheless, whether specified in Rogerian terms or as part of a more general stance of acceptance and warmth in the service of an effective therapeutic relationship, PR is an empirically supported (e.g., Farber, Suzuki, & Lynch,

2019), if underresearched and often misunderstood, aspect of psychotherapy. While we are quite sympathetic to Rogerian principles of psychotherapy, we are not exclusively devoted to this paradigm. In fact, consistent with the emerging research in the field, we do not believe that Rogers's three core conditions are inevitably necessary and sufficient to effect therapeutic change. Multiple other variables have been shown to be significant contributors to therapeutic progress (Norcross & Lambert, 2019; Norcross & Wampold, 2019). Our contention, rather, is that PR is of great importance in most psychotherapies; that it interacts with many relational and technical interventions; and that a comprehensive understanding of the nature, types, and consequences of PR may lead to greater mutual satisfaction in therapy as well as improved clinical outcomes.

In the next chapter, we review the research on the association of PR to treatment outcome, findings that provide support for our contention that all therapists should be adopting an attitude of PR in their clinical interactions.

2 POSITIVE REGARD AND TREATMENT OUTCOME

She had given him an astonishing gift, the gift of her interest.

–Brian Morton, *Starting Out in the Evening*

As subsequent chapters in this book document, clients and therapists alike believe strongly that the therapist's positive regard (PR) contributes substantially to the work of psychotherapy. But a critical question, especially for those therapists who believe deeply in the need for empirical support for their choice of interventions, is whether the therapist's provision of PR is significantly associated with treatment outcome. A brief historical perspective on efforts to understand whether and how psychotherapy "works" should provide some useful context to this question.

For many years after psychotherapy was invented, or at least systematized, by Freud, clinicians barely made attempts to assess its effectiveness. Practitioners of psychotherapy—and for the first half of the 20th century, that was essentially psychoanalysis—assumed that it worked, affirming the position of the major figures in the field. Skeptics or those wishing to scientifically

https://doi.org/10.1037/0000312-003
Understanding and Enhancing Positive Regard in Psychotherapy: Carl Rogers and Beyond, by B. A. Farber, J. Y. Suzuki, and D. Ort

investigate this form of healing were scoffed at. Freud's response, in the 1930s, to a researcher's attempts to investigate the concept of repression is a case in point:

> I have examined your experimental studies for the verification of the psycho-analytic assertions with interest. I cannot put much value on these confirma-tions because the wealth of reliable observations on which these assertions rest make them independent of experimental verification. (as cited by MacKinnon & Dukes, 1962, p. 703)

Clinical observations and case studies were seen as valid and sufficient methods of research, and successful treatments, per case study reports, were considered evidence of the effectiveness of the psychoanalytic method (Lees, 2005). Freud's power and status were such that, within the psychotherapeutic community, acceptance of the need to empirically validate psychotherapeutic claims of success was very slow in coming.

Gradually, though, the field of psychotherapy research took hold, and Carl Rogers was instrumental in this occurrence. At a time when such sentiments were rarely articulated, Rogers (1942) began calling for the field to be more open to and dependent on research: "Scientific progress in counseling can only take place as we have an adequate research analysis of adequate data. Up to the present time, we have never had adequate data" (p. 261). Among his many other notable accomplishments, Rogers was the first major psycho-therapeutic figure who insisted on testing the validity of his clinical ideas (Elliott & Farber, 2010). He was committed to making his clinical material available so that his therapeutic work could be independently evaluated. His (1942) book, *Counseling and Psychotherapy: Newer Concepts in Practice*, con-tains the first fully transcribed psychotherapy case ever published.

Despite Rogers's call for open examination of all facets of psychotherapy, the focus of this research for many years was not on the complex question of *how* therapy works but rather *whether* therapy works. Although early, methodologically flawed, and contentious attempts were made to prove that it does not work (e.g., Eysenck, 1952, 1966), researchers have clearly deter-mined that it does: Across multiple types of treatments, about 75% of those in therapy are better off than their nontreated counterparts (Lambert, 2013; Smith & Glass, 1980).

Whereas some research continues to investigate the overall effectiveness of psychotherapy, research in the last several decades has generally moved to the study of "what works," including investigation of client, therapist, and system variables associated with change (e.g., Bergin & Garfield, 1993; Lambert, 2003, 2013). Some studies of this type—and the ones that have garnered the most attention—have focused on investigating putative differences in the effectiveness of different brands of psychotherapy (e.g., cognitive behavior therapy [CBT] vs. psychodynamic therapy) for specific disorders (e.g., depression). Much to the chagrin of strong advocates of specific therapeutic traditions, the findings of these studies have indicated that, with few exceptions, there are no significant differences in treatment outcome as a function of therapeutic orientation (e.g., Wampold & Imel, 2015). These essentially null results have intensified efforts to identify which client, therapist, or treatment variables increase the probability of positive treatment effects. Even if all therapies are more or less equivalent in their effectiveness, surely there must be discrete factors that make a difference.

Most recently, this strand of research has focused on "relational variables," attempting to identify specific elements of the therapeutic relationship associated with therapeutic success. In this regard, John Norcross (2002, 2011; Norcross & Lambert, 2019; Norcross & Wampold, 2019) has edited several iterations of *Psychotherapy Relationships That Work*. Within each of these volumes, psychotherapy researchers who have studied a specific relational element have summarized the empirical work on that variable, culminating in a meta-analysis that combines the results of multiple studies to produce a single, overall statistic (e.g., Hedges's *g*) that indicates the overall strength of the association between that variable and therapeutic outcome. In the most recent two-set volume of this series (Norcross & Lambert, 2019; Norcross & Wampold, 2019), multiple aspects of the therapeutic relationship were found to be significantly associated with therapeutic outcome. Among these variables were the Rogerian conditions of PR, empathy, and genuineness, but there were several others, including the therapeutic alliance, therapist–patient collaboration, therapist–patient goal consensus, cultivating positive client expectations, managing therapist countertransference, and repairing alliance ruptures.

The most recent summary of the research linking PR to treatment outcome was published in 2019 (Farber, Suzuki, & Lynch, 2019)—and we go into detail about that study later in this chapter—but there have been multiple such attempts over the years. However, drawing firm conclusions from these efforts has proven difficult. The problems that often confound studies of complex psychological phenomena—small sample sizes, decades-old measures, lack of a standard operational definition of the concept or variable under study, conceptual overlap among related variables, and methodologically flawed research designs—have led to inconsistent findings in assessing the association of PR to outcome. Furthermore, the outcome measures used in virtually all of these studies assess symptom change, rather than increments in client self-esteem, self-acceptance, or relational satisfaction—the attitudes that therapist PR would more likely affect. Finally, as we noted in the Farber, Suzuki, and Lynch (2019) study,

> as the Rogerian influence on clinical practice has diminished in the last three to four decades—or, more accurately, has been incorporated into the psycho-therapeutic mainstream with little awareness or explicit acknowledgment (Farber, 2007)—empirical studies based on Rogerian concepts have also waned. (pp. 288–289)

In short, few studies on the effects of PR have been conducted in recent years.

MEASURES USED TO ASSESS THE ASSOCIATION BETWEEN POSITIVE REGARD AND TREATMENT OUTCOME

Most studies investigating the effects of therapist PR have used either the Barrett-Lennard Relationship Inventory (BLRI; Barrett-Lennard, 1964, 1978) or the Relationship Questionnaire (Truax & Carkhuff, 1967). The BLRI consists of 64 items across four domains—Empathic Understanding, Congruence, Level of Regard, and Unconditionality of Regard—the last two of which have been used in studies of PR. Level of Regard "is concerned in various ways with warmth, liking/caring, and 'being drawn toward'" (Barrett-Lennard, 1986, pp. 440–441). Positive items include "She respects me as a person," "I feel appreciated by her," and "She is friendly and warm toward me." Unconditionality of Regard represents stability of acceptance, "in the sense that it is not experienced as varying with or otherwise dependently linked to particular attributes of the person being regarded" (p. 443). Examples of positively worded items are "How much he likes or dislikes me is not altered by anything that I tell him about myself" and "I can (or could) be openly critical or appreciative of him without really making him feel any differently about me." As we noted previously, the Unconditionality subscale has declined in use as its psychometric properties have been called into question.

Truax, a collaborator of Rogers, developed two separate instruments for the measurement of Rogers's facilitative conditions. One was a set of scales to be used by raters either via live observations or audio recordings of sessions. There are five stages on the scale that measures Nonpossessive Warmth. At Stage 1, the therapist is "actively offering advice or giving clear negative regard" (Truax & Carkhuff, 1967, p. 60); at Stage 5, the therapist "communicates warmth without restriction. There is a deep respect for the patient's worth as a person and his rights as a free individual" (p. 66). (It is notable that actively offering advice is seen here as equivalent to communicating explicit negative regard.) The second instrument developed by Truax, the Relationship Questionnaire (Truax & Carkhuff, 1967), consists of 141 items that are to be marked "true" or "false" by the client. Among these items, 73 are keyed to the concept of Nonpossessive Warmth, including "He seems to like me no matter what I say to him," "He almost always seems very concerned about me," "He appreciates me," "I feel that he really thinks I am worthwhile," and "Whatever I talk about is OK with him." Thus, the items on this measure reflect a belief that PR (here designated as "Nonpossessive Warmth") consists of both an acceptance factor (what Rogers termed "Unconditionality") and an affirming/liking factor (what Barrett-Lennard termed "Level of Regard"). Many of the items on this measure are also keyed to the other two core conditions postulated by Rogers (empathy and genuineness), again reflecting their overlap.

Therapist PR has also been occasionally evaluated via measures designed for external coders to assess the strength of the alliance—for example, the Vanderbilt Psychotherapy Process Scale (VPPS; Suh et al., 1989). One of the subscales of the VPPS, Therapist Warmth and Friendliness, closely approximates the concept of PR. The specific therapist attributes rated in this subscale include "involvement" (the therapist's engagement in the patient's experience), "acceptance" (the therapist's ability to help the patient feel accepted), "warmth and friendliness," and "supportiveness" (the therapist's ability to bolster the patient's self-esteem, confidence, and hope). Therapist PR has also sometimes been measured through the use of structural analysis of social behavior (SASB; Benjamin, 1984), specifically through the dimension of Helping and Protecting. High scores on this dimension reflect the therapist's ability to teach or encourage a patient in a kind or positive manner.

The research literature has employed a wide range of outcome measures to assess the effectiveness of PR, ranging from specific symptom checklists to broader scales of client well-being, rated in some cases by the clients themselves and in other cases by treating clinicians or outside observers.

EARLY REVIEWS OF THE ASSOCIATION BETWEEN POSITIVE REGARD AND TREATMENT OUTCOME

The first comprehensive review of studies investigating the association of PR to clinical outcome was by Truax and Carkhuff (1967) in their book, *Toward Effective Counseling and Psychotherapy*. Among the many studies of Rogers's facilitative conditions they reviewed, 10 were used to draw conclusions about the distinctive effects of PR. Keeping in mind that both these researchers collaborated with Rogers and may have been vulnerable to experimenter bias, they reported that in eight of these studies, nonpossessive warmth (their preferred term) was significantly associated with therapeutic improvement.

The next iteration: Bergin and Garfield's (1971) first edition of *Handbook of Psychotherapy and Behavior Change* included a chapter by Truax and Mitchell (1971) that summarized the results of 12 studies that included nonpossessive warmth as a predictor variable. As above, they contended that the evidence was quite positive in regard to the association between warmth and therapeutic outcome, noting that there was a statistically significant relationship between this variable and a total of 34 specific outcome measures. Nevertheless, it is important to reiterate what others (e.g., Parloff et al., 1978) subsequently noted: that there are multiple ways of interpreting these data. For example, of 108 correlations noted in Truax and Mitchell's report, only 34 were reported as significantly positive. Although none of these correlations were significantly negative, relatively few (31.5%) were significantly positive.

In a follow-up review, K. M. Mitchell et al. (1977) evaluated 11 studies that investigated the association between PR (here again termed "nonpossessive warmth") and treatment outcome. The authors found that only four studies supported the proposition that higher levels of therapist-provided warmth led to better outcome. Their conclusion was more tempered than those of previous reviews: They suggested that warmth, empathy, and genuineness may all be related to client change but that "their potency and generalizability are not as great as some thought" (p. 483).

The following year, Orlinsky and Howard (1978) reviewed 23 studies, noting that in approximately two thirds of cases there was a significant positive association between therapist warmth and outcome, with the remaining studies yielding mostly null results. However, they added several caveats, notably that the uneven quality of the research made any firm conclusions suspect. Their summary, then, was also tempered: "If they [warmth and empathy] do not by themselves guarantee a good outcome, their presence probably adds significantly to the mix of beneficial therapeutic ingredients, and almost surely does no harm" (p. 293).

As part of a comprehensive review of process and outcome in psychotherapy, Orlinsky and Howard (1986) evaluated the separate effects of therapist support and therapist affirmation. They identified 11 studies focused on support, with a total of 25 discrete findings. Their conclusion was again modest: "Although 6 of the 25 are significantly positive findings and none are negative, more than three-quarters show a null association between specific therapist efforts to give support and patient outcome" (p. 326). In addition, they identified 94 findings about therapist affirmation (essentially, warmth, caring, and acceptance), noting that more than half (53%) demonstrated a significant association between affirmation and clinical outcome. However, the authors noted that "the proportion of positive findings is highest across all outcome categories when therapist warmth and acceptance are observed from the patient's process perspective" (p. 348). Whereas findings like this are problematic to methodologists, suggestive as they are of rater bias, they fit quite well with Rogers's contention that a meaningful assessment of PR (and the other facilitative conditions) can be made only by clients themselves.

In 1994, Orlinsky and colleagues studied *therapist affirmation*, described by the authors as a variable that includes aspects of acceptance, nonpossessive warmth, or positive regard. They found that 56% of the 154 results reviewed were positive and that, again, the findings based on patients' rating of the therapist's PR yielded a higher rate of positive therapeutic outcomes (65%). "Overall," Orlinsky et al. concluded, "nearly 90 findings indicate that therapist affirmation is a significant factor, but considerable variation in ES [effect size] suggests that the contribution of this factor to outcome differs according to specific conditions" (p. 326).

In their review of PR for the first edition of Norcross's *Psychotherapy Relationships That Work* (Norcross & Lambert, 2019; Norcross & Wampold, 2019)—the first assessment of this variable that included a meta-analysis— Farber and Lane (2002) primarily confirmed the results of several of the previous reviews. Of the 16 studies they analyzed, there was an essentially even split between positive and nonsignificant effects. That is, 49% (27/55) of all reported associations were significantly positive, and 51% (28/55) were nonsignificant. Consistent with previous reports, they found that when patients rated both PR and treatment outcome, a positive association between these variables was especially likely. In the second edition of Norcross's book on relational factors, Farber and Doolin (2011) analyzed a total of 18 studies, reporting an aggregate effect size (.27) that indicated that PR has a moderate positive association with psychotherapy outcomes.

THE MOST RECENT (2019) META-ANALYSIS

The most recent meta-analysis of research investigating the association between PR and psychotherapy outcomes (Farber, Suzuki, & Lynch, 2019) yielded a small-to-moderate overall positive relation between these variables, largely confirming the findings of earlier reviews and meta-analyses. Still, this iteration aimed to contextualize and deepen the analysis on a few fronts. We expanded the inclusion criteria to allow for studies investigating child, family, and group therapy, instead of just individual treatment with adult clients. Our search terms included *positive regard, unconditional positive regard, warmth, nonpossessive warmth, affirmation, therapist affirmation, validation,* and *acceptance*. In addition, in recognition of the fundamental interrelatedness of Rogers's three core conditions and the reality that in previous studies they were often measured collectively rather than individually, we included studies with "composite" predictor measures, primarily studies that grouped PR with empathy and/or genuineness. This decision was undertaken with the goal of assessing putative differences between the association of PR to treatment outcome when measured singly and when measured as part of a composite score.

With the expansion of these criteria, the meta-analysis comprised 369 effect sizes within 64 studies utilizing 3,528 unique participants, a notable increase from the data used in the analysis in 2011. Each effect size calculation took into account the sample size within each study to produce an unbiased estimate of the relation between PR and psychotherapy outcome. When using a statistical model that controlled for the fact that some data sets were used across multiple studies, the aggregate effect size was estimated at $g = .36$, amounting to a modest effect of PR on psychotherapy outcome. This result, although consistent with the moderate effect size ($r = .27$) found in Farber and Doolin's (2011) meta-analysis, is arguably a more robust indicator of PR's association to treatment outcome, both in terms of the significantly larger set of studies it draws from and with regard to the authors' reporting of *g*, a statistic that uses a more conservative metric than *r* in interpreting effect size.

As with all statistical analyses, it is essential to acknowledge that a variety of factors can contribute to findings that indicate that one variable (PR) is significantly associated with another (clinical outcome). In fact, we (Farber, Suzuki, & Lynch, 2019) found that when considered individually, multiple factors did contribute to the demonstrated significant association between PR and outcome. As we summarized,

> positive regard tends to have a more powerful association with psychotherapy outcome in individual therapy, in an outpatient setting, when therapy is performed by trainees, with clients presenting with mood or anxiety disorders (as opposed to severe mental illness), and when outcome is assessed via measures of global or overall symptomatology. (p. 308)

However, in the treatment room, these factors never operate in isolation, and one or more client, therapist, or treatment factors inevitably interact to influence outcomes. In recognition of this real-life complexity, the meta-analysis included a model combining (and controlling for the correlations among) all these significant moderators. The result: None of these demographic or treatment factors, including therapist theoretical orientation, was found to be a significant predictor of therapy outcome when considered in the broader subset of variables.

Another aspect of this meta-analysis that bears discussion is the finding that there was no significant difference in outcome when PR was assessed as a single factor versus when it was assessed as part of the triad of the facilitative conditions. This tends to confirm earlier theoretical and empirical literature that has indicated that PR, empathy, and genuineness are conflated. Whereas one could understand this as meaning that PR doesn't "need" the other two facilitative conditions to be effective in generating positive clinical outcome, the more clinically pragmatic hypothesis is that PR and the other two conditions blend. As we've noted previously, therapists' empathic reflections almost invariably feel positively regarding to clients; therapists who strive to be empathic are, in essence, conveying PR in attempting to understand their clients' experience. For PR to feel meaningful and have an impact on clients, this attitude would have to be conveyed authentically by therapists. Furthermore, as we also indicated earlier, the items on the BLRI scales that are most often used to assess the three facilitative conditions are not distinct; for example, several items that are keyed to the PR subscale are also keyed to the Empathy subscale. Stated otherwise, the way that PR is assessed, conveyed, and received often transcends nonjudgmental acceptance, becoming something on the order of a responsive/active listening mode, one that makes a significant difference in clinical outcome.

In sum, this meta-analysis, drawing comprehensively from the existing research, offers further evidence for Rogers's contention that empirical studies can offer support for the tenets of client-centered theory—in this case, the significant association between therapists' communication of PR and client treatment outcome.

POSITIVE REGARD, CULTURE, AND IDENTITY

The studies included in this most recent meta-analysis (Farber, Suzuki, & Lynch, 2019), though more diverse and comprehensive than in previous versions, were nonetheless culled from a limited pool. All but a few were published in English and sampled participants exclusively from American or European populations. Similarly, the existing body of research is grounded in U.S.-based scholarship, with predominantly White samples. As cultural and identity factors are increasingly acknowledged as extremely impactful on how we construct and understand ourselves and the world around us, some interrelated questions emerge: To what extent is our understanding of PR and its influence on the psychotherapy process a universal one? Can we assume that what we know about PR applies equally to therapy clients of different backgrounds? Do therapy clients universally experience PR as a meaningful ingredient in treatment? Is there significant culturally based variability in how clients expect or prefer to receive PR, beyond the variability we would expect from individual differences?

From one vantage point, the need for PR would seem to be universal, "a basic human need—pervasive and persistent" (Sanford, 2001, p. 74). Humans are profoundly social creatures, and social connection and affirmation are evolutionarily hardwired to be rewarding, even essential, to our survival and well-being. One imagines that in the context of a healing therapy relationship, this would be all the more true: that regardless of the client's sociocultural background or other demographic factors, a therapist's PR is an indispensable part of a client's ability to profit from therapeutic work.

The fact is, however, that there is little research that would substantiate or refute this supposition. Although the most recent meta-analysis (Farber, Suzuki, & Lynch, 2019) failed to find significant differences in the effects of PR on outcome as a function of several demographic factors, these results were based on a very limited number of studies. In particular, it was impossible to discern the effects of race or ethnicity or country of origin, or the dyadic matching of these variables, on the association of PR to clinical outcome. The therapists and patients in the included studies were overwhelmingly White and engaging in therapy in the United States. As we noted, this fact limited greatly our ability to identify possible effects for race and ethnicity.

Moreover, even if—broadly speaking—PR is a universal need, the specific forms that clients prefer and/or are most receptive to may vary substantially across cultures or demographic variables. Though scant, there is some research on these issues. As we discuss further in Chapter 6, we (Suzuki & Farber, 2016) found several variables that proved significant in clients' perceptions about the likelihood of certain types of PR occurring in their therapy or the affirming quality of different types of PR. For example, psychotherapy clients from countries other than the United States perceived boundary extensions in therapy, such as a therapist's hug, to be less indicative of PR than U.S.-based clients; clients identifying as non-White rated therapist statements that express support and caring—for example, "I'm glad you shared that with me"—as more affirming than White respondents; and self-identified LGBTQ respondents perceived therapist boundary extensions, including hugs or a hand on one's shoulder, as more affirming than did self-identified heterosexual respondents.

Another intriguing result was the finding that therapists of color were generally rated by their clients as more likely to explicitly express support and caring than their White counterparts. The meaning of this finding is open to multiple interpretations, but it is possible to imagine that therapists of color, working to actively counteract the harmful biases and stereotypes associated with their marginalized status, consciously or unconsciously feel compelled to put their clients at ease by being more explicitly affirming and warm in their interventions.

These limited findings are small examples of the myriad ways in which culture and identity-related variables in both the client and therapist shape the therapeutic relationship, including the communication and receipt of PR. Pedersen (1996) eloquently summarized this perspective:

> Although a loving, trusting and genuine relationship is important in all coun-
> seling, the way that rapport is established will reflect the complex and dynamic
> culture of each client. The right approach in one cultural context may well be
> the wrong approach in a different cultural context. (p. 236)

As noted earlier, Rogers posited that the therapist's attitude of PR is the fertile soil in which humans' inherent self-actualizing tendency, often stifled early in life by conditions of worth, can take root and flourish, resulting in an enhanced, more agentic sense of self. However, as Heine and colleagues (1999) pointed out, this understanding of how self and self-regard are constructed—through positive affirmations, by oneself and others, of the self as "good"—is fundamentally grounded in a Western perspective. Advancing a more ecumenical understanding, these authors argued that self-esteem arises from doing what is required by the cultural contexts within which one engages, emphasizing that self-regard can look quite different across cultures and that self-appraisals need not always be positive to promote self-esteem. They noted, for example, that

> Japanese criteria of self-hood support the individual in elaborating and focusing
> on potentially negative features of the self (i.e., to self-criticize) . . . this prac-
> tice of self-improvement serves to promote unity in relationships and simul-
> taneously affirms one's identity as an interdependent being committed to the
> shared values of the group. (p. 771)

If not as universally necessary and sufficient as Rogers had imagined, then surely therapist PR at least has some moderately salutary effect on the client's overall experience in therapy across cultural contexts? Again, the truth is that we lack sufficient evidence to support or refute this idea. Even as global practices and philosophies that predate modern psychotherapy by centuries have been co-opted and incorporated into mainstream Western approaches (e.g., mindfulness), the majority of psychotherapy approaches have been formalized in the West. Although treatment adaptation researchers and practitioners typically endeavor to ensure that treatments developed in a Western context are appropriately modified to increase cultural relevance, with rare exception (e.g., Freire et al., 2005) researchers have not reported the extent to which Rogers's core conditions have been part of treatment protocols nor the extent to which clients in these studies have responded to therapists' provision of empathy, genuineness, or PR. What goes unasked, of course, cannot be answered.

Heine and colleagues' (1999) work on cultural contrasts, as well as contemporary texts on multicultural counseling (e.g., Sue et al., 2019), serves to highlight the need for clinicians to be aware of assumptions they hold in their attempts to provide culturally informed care. And although our own research (e.g., Farber & Ort, 2021; Suzuki & Farber, 2016) and that of others have, somewhat surprisingly, pointed to only minimal differences in clients' preferences for, and responses to, PR as a function of demographic and identity-related factors, these issues have become more salient in recent times—and we imagine that new studies with greater numbers of millennial and Gen Z clients will find these factors to be increasingly significant.

Thus, in this moment (circa 2022) of growing awareness of ethnic, religious, racial, and gender-based biases, cultural and identity issues need to be primary concerns for clinicians when thinking about how to connect across difference—including how to convey and maintain an attitude of PR. That is, clinicians need to not only be aware of multiple aspects of their clients' identities but also become more fully aware of their own culturally learned and internalized assumptions—understanding how their own particular perspectives and blind spots mediate the work of becoming more culturally sensitive, including providing appropriate forms and degrees of PR.

White clinicians, for example, may attempt to understand the perspectives and lived experiences of clients identifying as BIPOC (Black, Indigenous, and other people of color) or otherwise dissimilar from themselves, and this may well be clinically meaningful and helpful in establishing a foundation for culturally sensitive therapeutic work (e.g., Sue et al., 2019). But rather than focusing exclusively on understanding the meaning of their clients' racial or other identity-related experiences—a well-intentioned action but one that can unwittingly evoke the alienating age-old question "How does it feel to be a problem?" (DuBois, 1903/2019)—they might choose to become curious about how their own Whiteness (or another component of their identity) affects their ability to demonstrate PR in the treatment room (e.g., Baima & Sude, 2020).

HOW MIGHT POSITIVE REGARD LEAD TO GOOD CLINICAL OUTCOME?

To the extent that the consensus among the reviews of PR's effectiveness is that there is a moderate and significant association between this variable and treatment outcome, how might we account for these results? What are the mechanisms by which PR leads to beneficial clinical results? There are several compelling ideas as to how PR contributes to positive therapeutic effects.

In a paper ("Experiences in Communication") he wrote in 1964 that was later republished in his book *A Way of Being,* Rogers (1980) provided his most personal and detailed attempt to explain how PR makes a difference in clients' lives. On a broad level, he contended that this therapeutic attitude lessens the hold of early experiences of conditions of worth—that clients begin to believe, and increasingly live in accordance with the belief, that they are essentially good and worthy of their own respect and that of others. By recounting instances in his own life when he felt "overcome by feelings of worthlessness and despair," he delved further than usual into how others' PR made a difference:

> When someone really hears you without passing judgment on you, without trying to take responsibility for you, without trying to mold you, it feels damn good! At these times it has released the tension in me. It has permitted me to bring out the frightening feelings, the guilts, the despair, the confusions that have been a part of my experiences. When I have been listened to and when I have been heard, I have been able to perceive my world in a new way and to go on. It is astonishing how elements that seem insoluble when someone listens, how confusions that seem irremediable turn into relatively clear flowing streams when one is heard. (Rogers, 1980, p. 12)

Most fundamentally, then, and consistent with Rogers's thoughts, the essential effect of the therapist's support and acceptance is the client's greater self-acceptance and self-prizing; these qualities have been termed *unconditional positive self-regard* (Patterson & Joseph, 2006). The therapist's dependable provision of PR leads to the client's greater belief in themself, including the felt sense that one can tolerate life's inevitable disappointments, pain, and setbacks more effectively. One could conceptualize this, as well, in terms of a client's increase in self-esteem and sense of agency or, to use Frank's (1961) term, remoralization. No matter the terms used, clients who have struggled to believe in their own worth begin to feel otherwise, as a result of the therapist's consistent acceptance, support, and caring. As Cain (2010) remarked,

> As clients realize that they are seen for whom they *are* and valued, they may revise the views they have of themselves in more positive directions and become

more self-accepting. Previously introjected conditions of worth from significant others (e.g., "I am acceptable if . . .") are counteracted and reduced as clients experience and absorb the therapist's regard for them, as well as the regard from others that was previously dismissed because it was felt to be undeserved. (p. 83)

In a similar vein, clients who feel their thoughts and feelings accepted by a valued other—their therapist—can shift their locus of evaluation from external sources to what Rogers (1959) deemed an internal locus of evaluation. This is one of the great benefits of PR within the context of person-centered therapy, one stemming from an essential attitude, toward clients, of "I believe that you have within yourself the capacity to grow and lead your own life in accord with your own feelings, needs, and values, and I will support your growth in this direction." Clients exposed to this attitude begin to act more consistently in accord with their own needs, looking less frequently and/or intensely to external sources to validate their choices. As Cain (2010) noted, "making choices based on one's own beliefs, values, and senses may be experienced as more risky but may also result in feelings of pride, confidence, and self-reliance" (p. 24).

Importantly, too, as clients become more self-accepting, they tend to become more accepting of others and better able to negotiate mutually satisfying personal relations. As some of the interviewees in one of our studies (Suzuki, 2018) indicated, a therapist's PR can lead to increased trust in, and comfort around, others. PR, like empathy, can also lessen one's sense of aloneness in the world; it partially attenuates existential isolation and meaninglessness. Individuals to whom PR is consistently addressed feel a greater sense of respect and value and can more confidently express their own needs and feelings within relationships.

Lietaer (2001) provided another perspective on the mutative properties of PR: "As a result of the unconditional acceptance of the therapist, the client gradually feels safe enough to explore himself more deeply, to face aspects that up to that moment had been too threatening or too shameful" (p. 90). Lietaer's idea here points to a common element among person-centered, psychoanalytic, and behavioral and CBT therapists: that in their own style and consistent with their theoretical tenets, practitioners from diverse orientations help clients find ways in which they can accept previously unexplored or disavowed aspects of themselves. Classical psychoanalytic practitioners, via their adoption of the attitudes of neutrality, anonymity, and abstinence (the so-called analytic triad), facilitate clients' ability to pursue the "fundamental rule" of saying whatever is on their mind. In a somewhat though clearly not identical manner, the acceptance, affirmation, and nonjudgmental manner of person-centered practitioners (and contemporary relationally oriented psychodynamic therapists) provides the conditions for their clients to safely discuss and accept previously unacceptable aspects of the self. Providing some empirical support for this position, Velasquez and Montiel (2018) analyzed 31 sessions of Rogers's work with clients, concluding that his attitude of PR promoted clients' "discourse elaboration." Behavioral and CBT therapists, especially those that employ mentalization/mindfulness techniques, also find ways for their clients to feel safe or relaxed enough to try out new behaviors, thoughts, or feelings.

Our sense is that PR can indeed facilitate a client's willingness to share aspects of themselves with a trusted, accepting therapist. But we believe, too, based on our interviews with clients and the clinical literature, that this often occurs in the context of the provision of all of Rogers's facilitative conditions or, from a broader pantheoretical perspective, within the context of an effective therapeutic alliance. Empirical work on factors affecting patient disclosure provides some indirect support for this overall hypothesis: Patients do disclose more when they feel the alliance is stronger (Farber, 2006).

Individuals outside the therapy room also tend to disclose more when they feel safer, accepted, and cared for. In her recent best-selling book, *Little Fires Everywhere*, Celeste Ng (2017) offered an excellent illustration of how a small act of caring can create a safe enough space for someone to unburden herself of long-held secrets:

> In her experience, when someone tried to do something for her, it came from either pity or distance, but this simple gesture [of being offered a homemade sandwich] felt like what it was: a small kindness, with no strings attached. When she had finished the last bite of sandwich, she licked butter from her fingers and looked up.
> "So you want to hear what happened?" she asked, and the whole story emerged. (p. 75)

Conversely, in his best-selling memoir, *My Struggle: Book 1*, the Norwegian author Karl Ove Knausgaard (2009/2013) recounted how the presence of his terrifying, judgmental father restricted the scope of family conversation:

> If he [my father] was outside the house or down in his study, we chatted as loudly and freely and with as many gesticulations as we liked; if he was on his way up the stairs we automatically lowered our voices and changed the topic of conversation, in case we were talking about something we assumed he might consider unseemly; if he came into the kitchen we stopped altogether, sat there as stiff as pokers, to all outward appearances sunk in concentration over the food; on the other hand, if he retired to the living room we continued to chat, but more warily and more subdued. (p. 17)

In short, even as just one part of a constellation of relational factors, PR likely contributes to the sense of safety often necessary for deeply personal disclosures. In turn, such disclosures offer multiple pathways toward healing.

One, noted previously, is the opportunity to accept aspects of oneself that have been difficult to acknowledge. Other benefits of disclosing include feeling closer to one's therapist and thus experiencing oneself as capable of greater intimacy with another; becoming more self-aware and able to see oneself and others through a more complex lens; enhancing one's feeling of being genuine, of living authentically; and experiencing great relief from the often-formidable burden of keeping painful thoughts or feelings to oneself (Farber, Blanchard, & Love, 2019). In regard to this last point: Shame, often such a toxic emotion, may become attenuated as a client reveals hard truths or discomforting experiences to a fully accepting, nonjudgmental therapist. "I had the feeling that the counsellor accepts these feelings, and then these feelings disappeared" (Timulák & Lietaer, 2001, p. 68).

Another pathway by which PR facilitates good clinical outcome is through its salutary effects on the therapeutic relationship, itself a variable that has been shown to be significantly associated with effective treatment (Flückiger et al., 2018). Clients whom we interviewed about their experience with PR in their therapy consistently endorsed the idea that PR strengthens the relationship, lessening the likelihood of damaging ruptures and enabling them to feel emotionally closer to their therapist and disclose more freely (Suzuki, 2018).

Many of these presumptive effects of PR are consistent with how theorists and researchers view the clinical effects of empathy. This should not be surprising, given the widely held idea that a therapist's PR is often expressed through empathic resonance with their client. Therapists' empathy has been thought to increase clients' self-worth, facilitate greater awareness of experience, enhance self-compassion, regulate affect, attenuate self-criticism, and strengthen the therapeutic relationship (Bohart & Greenberg, 1997; Gelso, 2019; Watson et al., 2014, 2020).

In sum, research has provided credible empirical evidence that therapists' PR, as a stand-alone component or as one element of Rogers's three core attitudinal conditions considered together, is a clinically effective relational variable and one that works across multiple theoretical orientations. Meta-analytic results, combined with the clinical views of prominent theorists (including Rogers), findings from research on empathy, and data obtained from client interviews, indicate that therapist-provided PR reduces symptomatology, enhances the therapeutic relationship, attenuates shame, and promotes multiple aspects of personal growth and competency, including self-regulatory capacities. It is not a panacea, though no intervention or attitude or medication is. All therapies tend to have the same rate of success (Wampold & Imel, 2015), and many patients, particularly those who have suffered especially traumatic childhoods, will suffer clinical relapses and need years of treatment to keep them on a relatively even keel. Nevertheless, for most patients across all mainstream therapies, PR is an effective clinical tool—and one with few, if any, downsides. Although certain theoretical models long resisted adopting PR as part of their overall clinical approach, it is a positive development and a win for clients that virtually all therapies now emphasize the importance of multiple aspects of the patient–therapist relationship, including PR.

In the next two chapters, we examine how Rogers's original understanding of PR has been modified by those within and without the person-centered community, providing new ways for therapists to adopt and enhance this fundamental attitude in the service of their clients.

3 RECONCEPTUALIZING POSITIVE REGARD

Let Me Count the Ways

Don't go changing to try to please me . . . I'll take you just the way you are.
—Billy Joel, "Just the Way You Are"

Carl Rogers was not the first historical figure to believe in the value and import of treating others with respect, acceptance, warmth, and attentiveness. One can find strains in the ancient writings of Buddhism (four great virtues: equanimity or acceptance, compassion, lovingkindness, and sympathetic joy), Islam (*rahmah*, understood as compassion and mercy), Christianity (Jesus: "Judge not"), and Judaism ("Judge everyone favorably"). One can even find strands in the 1936 self-help book by Dale Carnegie, *How to Win Friends and Influence People*, a work that has sold over 30 million copies.

However, in one sense, Carl Rogers was an original. At a time when psychoanalysis was essentially a hegemonic force in the therapeutic universe, he understood that there were other ways of attending to and helping those with psychological concerns. It was a powerful new way of helping, one that has had enormous resonance within nearly every contemporary form of psychotherapy,

https://doi.org/10.1037/0000312-004
Understanding and Enhancing Positive Regard in Psychotherapy: Carl Rogers and Beyond, by B. A. Farber, J. Y. Suzuki, and D. Ort

even the psychodynamic community that was once so hostile to his message. And yet, no therapy, no theory, is truly sui generis.

Rogers was not the first prominent therapist to believe the relationship was instrumental in effecting change—Otto Rank, a member of Freud's inner circle and a maverick psychoanalyst in his own right, is a better candidate for that honor. As noted earlier, Rank's (1936/1978) sense was that classical psychoanalysis too often denied or minimized the importance of the therapeutic relationship; he believed that effective therapy needed to be experiential, relational, and focused on the here and now. There is even evidence that Freud himself acted far more in accord with the principles of what would later be deemed client-centered, humanistic, or contemporary relational psychotherapy than he acknowledged and that these actions and this attitude on his part may have had a far greater effect on the progress and outcome of his patients than he or his followers realized:

> When Freud followed these [psychoanalytic] rules his patients did not make progress. His well-known published cases are failures . . . in contrast are patients like Kardiner and others—cases he never wrote or publicly spoke about—all of whom found their analyses very helpful. With these patients, what was curative was not neutrality, abstinence, or interpretations of resistance, but a more open and supportive relationship, interpretations that fit their unique experiences, empathy, praise, and the feelings that they were liked by their analyst. (Breger, 2009, p. 105)

Moreover, despite Freud's austere recommendations for clinical practice and his view that all kindness on the part of therapists could be considered seductive (Storr, 2001)—that is, inevitably exercised for unconscious ulterior motives—he occasionally gave gifts and loaned patients books, chatted with them about personal matters, and on at least one occasion comforted a distressed patient by momentarily taking her hand (Momigliano, 1987).

Nevertheless, Freud and—even more so—his immediate followers tended, in their writings, to proscribe any deviation from psychoanalytic dicta, holding fast to the belief in the analytic posture of neutrality (nondirective, evenly suspended attention), abstinence (nongratification of patient needs, resisting the temptations of conveying warmth and support), and anonymity (nondisclosure of personal information). Those who deviated from Freudian orthodoxy and the significance of these conditions (or of the centrality of the Oedipus complex), including Rank, Ferenczi, and Jung, were disparaged and ultimately banished from Freud's inner circle. It was Rogers, influenced by Rank, who offered a very different perspective on the way that therapists should be with their clients, including the need for therapists to be genuine, emotionally (not just intellectually) empathic, and positively regarding. From a Rogerian perspective, these were characteristics for therapists to strive for, not hide from. And whereas

Rank's ideas were essentially scorned or ignored within the psychoanalytic community, Rogers's ideas came to serve as the foundation for a new and highly influential form of psychotherapy, one that has greatly changed the way that all therapies think about the nature and importance of the therapeutic relationship.

But Rogers's take on the mutative conditions of therapy, especially positive regard (PR), underwent some changes over the years. In the books on adult psychotherapy that Rogers (1942, 1951) wrote or coedited (Rogers & Dymond, 1954) prior to his 1957 journal article ("The Necessary and Sufficient Conditions of Therapeutic Personality Change"), he never used the term "positive regard," referring instead to "acceptance" and occasionally "warmth." Furthermore, once the term "positive regard" was introduced in Standal's (1954) dissertation and then incorporated into Rogers's 1957 article, Rogers continually redefined PR—and others did, as well. As with virtually all philosophies, religious dicta, political platforms, and social science theories, original tenets undergo changes as followers subject the founders' assumptions and beliefs to critical analyses and their own interpretations. Contemporary relational dynamic psychotherapy shares some assumptions with classical psychoanalysis but is also significantly different (e.g., in terms of the former's emphasis on the value of the therapeutic relationship, including prudent degrees of self-disclosure; Wachtel, 2008); similarly, emotion-focused therapy draws on the tenets of Perls and gestalt therapy (e.g., a focus on here-and-now feelings) but is also strikingly different (e.g., has a more humanistic tone; Greenberg, 2002). Similarly, Rogers's original ideas about what constituted PR—essentially an acceptance of the client that is optimally invariant ("unconditional") and contains elements of warmth and caring and even nonpossessive love—soon began to be reinterpreted.

There have been three significant sources of modification and reinterpretation of PR. One group of interpreters was (and still is) composed of adherents to a client-centered (now person-centered) perspective on human development and psychotherapy. Much like Freud's followers, those who have essentially aligned themselves with Rogers's theories have nevertheless had their own ideas about the nature and role of the core principles within this system, ideas that do not perfectly correspond to Rogers's ideas. For example, several figures within the client- or person-centered tradition (e.g., Bozarth, 1996, 1998, 2013; Lietaer, 1984; Mearns, 1994; Wilkins, 2010) have differed from Rogers in regard to the associations among PR, empathy, and congruence; the relative primacy of these conditions; and/or the legitimacy of a more active or theoretically eclectic stance in providing PR to clients. Furthermore, as Bozarth (2013) noted, "the fact remains that there is a substantially different view of UPR in post-classical therapies in relation to Rogers' theory of therapy" (p. 184). By this, he meant that there are several forms of therapy, including focusing-experiential therapy (Gendlin, 1978) and emotion-focused therapy (Greenberg, 2016; Johnson, 2019), that have appropriated aspects of person-centered therapy (e.g., in terms of the primacy of the relationship and a focus on here-and-now feelings) but have not retained traditional views of how unconditional positive regard (UPR) should be provided. Instead of an emphasis on acceptance, many of these newer, hybrid therapies have allowed or promoted more explicit means (e.g., validating statements) for therapists to be positively regarding.

A second group consists of those outside the person-centered tradition who, while not typically employing the specific words "positive regard," have nonetheless written about overlapping concepts (e.g., Linehan's ideas about "validation" and "radical acceptance," Kohut's ideas about "mirroring" and "empathic attunement") in ways that have influenced the perception in the wider therapeutic community about what is meant by PR. Whereas Rogers, as early as 1951, took pains to note that being "supportive" should not translate to therapists being "supportive or approving in the superficial sense" (p. 71)—meaning they should not be actively affirming or complimentary—those outside the client- or person-centered tradition have not always adhered to this sense of what support or affirmation should look like. And neither did Rogers, as we detail below.

A third group responsible for redefining the nature of PR has been psychotherapy researchers. Within this subset, some have devised measures and/or conducted factor analytic studies that have modified the number of factors constituting PR. For example, several researchers (e.g., Barrett-Lennard, 1978; Gurman, 1977) have suggested that PR consists not of just two factors—one reflective of acceptance/caring/warmth and another reflective of unconditionality—but also an additional, third factor: nondirectivity. This factor harkens back to the early days of client-centered therapy, when it was typically called "nondirective therapy" (Raskin, 1948) and emphasized the need for the clinician only to follow the client's direction and to believe in the client's ability to make choices for their life. Adding yet another possibility, Eckert et al. (1988) studied PR through assessing four putative features: warmth, respect, acceptance, and interest. According to their findings, warmth and respect are the more relevant factors in the process of symptom change, particularly among clients with the most severe symptoms. Other researchers (e.g., Farber & Ort, 2021; Suzuki & Farber, 2016) have conducted studies of PR that have broadened the domain of what Rogers suggested falls under the rubric of PR. They have done so by designing new measures of PR that include items (e.g., overt support or compliments) that transcend Rogers's beliefs about what constitutes this attitude.

In this chapter, we review the ways that theorists adopting the person-centered approach (PCA) have criticized and, in some instances, extended Rogers's views on the nature of PR. In the next chapter, we turn to the ways in which theorists outside the person-centered tradition have reformulated or appropriated Rogers's ideas into concepts that resemble, though are not identical to, traditional definitions of PR. In Chapters 6 and 7, we present research, based on the perspectives of clients and therapists, that offers new ways of thinking about the ways in which PR may be understood and adopted by practitioners.

HAS POSITIVE REGARD GOTTEN MORE OVERTLY POSITIVE? AND IF SO, WHY?

Before delving more deeply into the divergent ways of conceptualizing PR offered by those associated with the PCA, we briefly speculate what might have happened had Rogers stayed with the term "acceptance" (used throughout his 1951 book, *Client-Centered Therapy*) rather than adopting Standal's term "positive regard." One could argue that the apparent drift toward active affirmation as a component of PR, including Rogers's use of the word "prizing" and even his occasional and surprising use of compliments (e.g., his oft-quoted statement to Gloria, in their filmed demonstrations interview [Shostrom, 1965], that she looked "like a pretty nice daughter"), might never have occurred.

This argument is predicated on the assumption that the phrase itself, with its inclusion of the word "positive," somehow provided the impetus for adopting an attitude that included greater latitude for greater degrees of support and encouragement and even some semblance of overt approval. "Positive regard" does seem to imply something more affectively loaded or interpersonally embracing than "acceptance." On the other hand, well before Standal's (1954) dissertation, from where Rogers appropriated the term "positive regard" (and "conditions of worth"), Rogers (1942) used the phrase "warmth and responsiveness on the part of the counselor" (p. 88), allowing for and even suggesting that a significant emotional component could and should be a part of the therapist's general acceptance of, and regard for, clients.

Thus, while it is tempting to believe that Rogers's adoption of the term "positive regard" as one of the central features of his theoretical model changed the way he and others defined this attitude, we believe it more likely that the modifications that ensued—and these have tended to be more gradual than radical in the direction of greater degrees of active or explicit affirmation—were made in response to cultural changes in the United States. The transformations made to the boundaries of PR were consistent with the movement in the mid- to late-1960s and thereafter toward greater and more overt manifestations of intimacy, including emotional (and sometimes physical) intimacy. Often termed the "human potential movement," individuals were encouraged, and sometimes taught, to express their feelings openly and honestly and to search for and appreciate the good in others. Rogers was instrumental in this reshaping of the culture. He moved to California, the epicenter of this movement, in 1963; established the Center for the Studies of the Person in 1968; and spent most of the rest of his life there (La Jolla), writing, lecturing, leading workshops, and participating in encounter groups. He spoke of encounter or sensitivity groups—of face-to-face open disclosures of feelings and emotional reactions between participations—as "the most significant social invention of the century" (Fehr, 2003, p. 22). All therapeutic approaches are a product of the zeitgeist, inevitably responding to cultural changes and needs (e.g., Yassky, 1979). In the case of client-centered therapy, an approach so tied to a single, enormously influential figure, Rogers's immersion in these new cultural trends was certain to have an impact on the nature and interpretations of his basic theoretical tenets.

In short, our sense is that the inevitable modifications made by Rogers and by those in his orbit in conceptualizing PR (and the other facilitative conditions), catalyzed in part by the significant cultural changes of the 1960s, led to a greater general allowance of a stronger, more overt affirmative dimension as part of an overall PR attitude toward clients. Whereas PR always included a "warmth" component, this part of the definition now seemed to be accentuated, sometimes to the point of explicit indications of the therapist's approval, caring, and/or praise. Let's again take Rogers's words to Gloria (Shostrom, 1965) as an example of what we are suggesting. Rogers could have chosen to respond to Gloria's remark ("Gee, I'd like you for my father") with simple acceptance, something on the order of "Yes, I understand that." Or, he could have added some more warmth or emotional content to that comment, something on the order of, "I can sense how much you mean that"—which would have been more typical of his way of expressing PR. In fact, though, he chose to be quite affirming, even flattering: "You look to me like a pretty nice daughter."

Whereas one could view this as an anomalous response, an exception to the theoretical prescriptions of how PR should be conveyed, it was not the only time Rogers responded in this fashion. D. Larson (personal communication, April 9, 2020) related a story about speaking with Rogers several years after his filmed interview with Gloria. Larson, curious as most are after having seen this work, asked Rogers whether there was any postinterview follow-up between the two of them. Some of what Rogers told Larson was already well known—for example, that Gloria corresponded with Rogers on multiple occasions and regretted her favorable postinterview filmed comments to the producer of the video (Shostrom) about her work with Perls. But Rogers, in his conversation with Larson, added a piece to this now well-documented story: that Gloria, having been diagnosed with cancer (leukemia) many years later, reached out to Rogers, describing her dilemma as to whether she should opt for treatment that would likely prolong her life or forgo treatment in the service of better quality of life. Said Rogers to Gloria during that conversation, "I can't make that decision [as to whether you should choose treatment] for you, but I know that whatever choice you make, it will be a courageous one" (D. Larson, personal communication, April 9, 2020). This is remarkably moving and, of course, sad—Gloria died shortly thereafter at the age of 46. But this dialogue also illustrates the fact that Carl Rogers did sometimes go beyond acceptance, beyond nondirectiveness, to offer personal words of admiration. Rogers also loaned money and occasionally provided cigarettes to one of the hospitalized patients he was seeing as part of the Wisconsin project (Bozarth, 1996) and occasionally held hands with clients who requested this of him (e.g., Whiteley, 1980).

Lietaer and Gundrum's (2018) categorization of Rogers's responses to clients over his career includes other examples of Rogers being actively supportive and/or complimentary—for example, "You have quite a gift for saying things" (p. 290), "I would just bet that a lot of these people think that's the best speech they've heard in a long, long time" (p. 281), "I feel it's been a privilege to see an older person who is young" (p. 296), "I appreciate being with you" (p. 296), and "I thank you for your courage in coming here" (p. 296). Their system of categorizing Rogers's responses did not include a category for positive regard per se. The category they used was termed "confirmation, support," and per their calculations, the percentage of Rogers's responses that fit under this category rose from 0.3 in years 1950 to 1957 while he was in Chicago to 1.5 in years 1965 to 1986 while he was in La Jolla and elsewhere in California.

According to Lietaer and Gundrum (2018),

> Rogers almost never confirms or reassures the client explicitly in separate response segments. . . . In our opinion, this does not mean that Rogers is not supporting the client. We think he communicates his confirming attitude mainly indirectly through his receptive and empathic openness to whatever the client communicates. (p. 301)

But they also hedged their bets somewhat, because they also noted in their quite-detailed analysis of Rogers's responses that, over time, he adopted a more flexible response style, one that reflected the "specific momentary needs of each client" and involved a "freer use of self," more directivity, and a greater shift to a more personal "I–Thou stance" (p. 305).

To return, then, to our original question of whether PR has gotten more overtly positive: No, if our answer is embedded within the perspective of Rogers's theory, one still embraced by traditionalists within the person-centered community and one that privileges acceptance and strongly discourages explicit indications of approval or any evaluation; but yes, if our answer is based on more contemporary views and clinical practice.

CHANGES AND CHALLENGES WITHIN THE PERSON-CENTERED COMMUNITY

Many of the innovations in thinking about PR post Carl Rogers are contained in Bozarth and Wilkins's (2001) edited book on UPR. Across 18 chapters, many of the most prominent figures within the person-centered community affirmed, revised, and/or offered personal reflections on Rogers's ideas about this facilitative condition.

At the outset, the editors stated their own beliefs about UPR:

> In terms of theory and our own experience, we understand the client's perception of unconditional positive regard (UPR) to be the active facilitator of constructive personality change . . . we have both asserted that unconditional positive regard is the curative factor in person-centered therapy. (Bozarth & Wilkins, 2001, p. vii)

Consistent with Rogers, they believed that therapists' provision of UPR is so important because it counters previously experienced conditions of worth, experiences that have inhibited the development of the "individual's internal valuing system," thus preventing "free and full functioning" and leading to a state of incongruence (Bozarth & Wilkins, 2001, p. ix). However, several authors contributing chapters to this book challenged or attempted to modify Rogers's ideas. Some of the questions they raised are noted next, along with some questions and challenges noted more recently by those aligned with the person-centered tradition, and our responses to these ideas.

Can a Therapist's Confrontations Be Considered Within the Domain of Positive Regard?

Lietaer's (1984) oft-cited paper "Unconditional Positive Regard: A Controversial Basic Attitude in Client-Centered Therapy" was originally published in 1980 (in Dutch), subsequently reprinted as a chapter in an edited book (Levant & Shlien, 1984), and revised for inclusion in Bozarth and Wilkins's

2001 book under the revised title "Unconditional Acceptance and Positive Regard" (Lietaer, 2001). For the most part, Lietaer accepted Rogers's ideas about UPR. Congruence and unconditionality (absolute acceptance, an "evaluative moratorium") are, for Lietaer, the foundational principles underlying client-centered therapy. As we noted briefly in the first chapter, Lietaer (2001) contended that these two ways of being constitute "a basic attitude of openness"—openness to oneself (congruence) and openness to all facets of one's client (unconditionality). Acceptance, wrote Lietaer (2001), "enables evolution of frozen aspects of ourselves" (p. 90).

Lietaer (2001) also argued for including that third component (nondirectivity) in any attempt to understand UPR, a component he suggested is most closely approximated by the term "client-centeredness." By this, he meant that a therapist conveying PR—at least within the client- or person-centered tradition—necessarily respects the right of clients to live in accord with their values, principles, and needs, assiduously refraining from imposing the therapist's own values or frame of reference into therapy sessions. Clients' needs regarding the pace of therapy, the issues discussed, and new directions taken must be totally respected.

Lietaer's most significant deviation from classical client-centered thought is that he advocated for a more active form of UPR, even considering some types of confrontation as falling within the acceptable bounds of this concept. Even though Lietaer's (2001) use of the term "confrontation" in the quote below is better thought of as providing honest and accurate feedback to the client, it still extends the concept well beyond what Rogers and traditional client-centered theorists described. One can see how PR, or at least its unconditionality strand, is slipping into something broader here—something that now allows any honest thoughts from the therapist, so long as they contain elements of empathy, congruence, and a nonjudgmental attitude, to be considered within the domain of PR.

> For confrontation does not in any way mean that I reject my client as a person or that I stop trying to understand his experience. First of all, not every confrontation stems from feelings of irritation. For instance, I might confront my client with his strengths and possibilities, or with facets of his experience that are hardly conscious, or even with positive feelings on my part. In addition, there are of course confrontations that have to do with difficulties in our relationship. Such moments of confrontation stand the best chance of having a constructive effect when at the same time I can experience and communicate a deep feeling of engagement. (Lietaer, 2001, p. 100)

Thus, in Lietaer's (2001) view, interpretations, accurate feedback, therapist disclosures of here-and-now feelings, and even attempts to resolve alliance ruptures can all be considered under the large umbrella of PR—if they also reflect the principles of Rogers's facilitative conditions. Lietaer invoked Eugene Gendlin—a student of Rogers who later became noted for his work on experiential "focusing"—as an ally in this expanded view. UPR, wrote Gendlin (1970),

> includes our expressions of dismay and even anger, but always in the context of both of us knowing we are seeking to meet each other warmly and honestly as people, exactly at the point at which we each are and feel. (p. 549)

By extension, then, a therapist who shares their feelings with the client—countertransferential thoughts or feelings in psychodynamic terms—is providing PR if they do so in a caring and genuine fashion.

We are reminded of Perls's work with Gloria (Shostrom, 1965) in a session immediately following Rogers's time with this volunteer client. Close to the end of their interview, Gloria expressed her frustration with his harsh and even demeaning comments to her: "I'm mad at you . . . I feel like you're not recognizing me at all, Dr. Perls, not a bit." In response, Perls said, "I respect you so much as a human being that I refuse to accept the phony part of yourself." Watching the interview, it's difficult to conclude that Perls's treatment of Gloria falls within the category of PR. Yet, if we expand the domain of PR in a manner consistent with Lietaer, then even Perls's no-holds-barred assessment and treatment of his client, so long as it seemingly includes a genuine respect for her, can be considered a legitimate manifestation of this general attitude. One could say much the same about the often-acerbic clinical manner of Albert Ellis, a manner that many would struggle to perceive as positively regarding yet can be seen as respectful in terms of his unflinching honesty about his clients' self-defeating patterns. In contrast to Lietaer's views, we do not believe that all therapist interventions that are seemingly genuine, including confrontations, are necessarily positively regarding. Indeed, consistent with one of Rogers's (1957) postulates, we believe that any therapist communication, whether made from a place of genuineness or not, cannot be considered as positively regarding if not experienced as such by the client. But we do believe that there are multiple ways of conveying PR, some of which go beyond Rogers's original ideas.

We revisit this issue in a later chapter when we review the findings of a large-scale survey (Suzuki & Farber, 2016) of clients' views about what they consider to be positively regarding. The "spoiler" here is that, at least from clients' perspectives, PR can indeed stem from therapists' active interventions and explicit words of encouragement.

Can Positive Regard Be "Faked"?

In his own chapter within his coedited book, Wilkins (2000/2001) raised several points about UPR. He was ambivalent about accepting Lietaer's sense that confrontation and providing accurate feedback are "allowable" as aspects of UPR. On the one hand, he aligned himself with Bozarth (1998) in the belief that these kinds of interactions are not benign, because they lead to a "shift in emphasis from trusting the client's experience towards trusting the 'expertise' of the therapist" (Bozarth, 1998, p. 85). On the other hand, Wilkins contended that if UPR is experienced by the client, then challenge and confrontation on the part of the therapist may be appropriate and useful. His position seems to be that as long as the therapist allows clients to pursue their own agenda in therapy, such that they feel unconditionally accepted, the therapist is allowed a wide latitude in expressing PR.

Wilkins (2000/2001) also contended that "because it depends on the attitude individuals hold toward themselves, unconditional positive regard is the hardest therapeutic attitude to develop" (p. 42). By this, he meant that therapists must accept themselves—everything that "bubbles up in them," to use one of Rogers's favorite phrases—in order to effectively and genuinely provide PR to others. Therapists can neither empathize with nor accept disparate facets of another until and unless they accept these aspects in themselves. Wilkins's assumption here is consistent with psychoanalytic dicta that psychoanalysts cannot effectively perform the work unless they have been analyzed and thus reduced or minimized their own "blind spots." Wilkins may be right. Although therapists' personal therapy has not been consistently shown to correlate with client outcome, there are data that suggest that personal therapy has a positive effect on the ability of therapists to offer Rogers's facilitative conditions (Macran & Shapiro, 1998).

However, Wilkins (2000/2001) also wrote that UPR "cannot be effectively faked" (p. 42), a proposition that has neither been empirically proven nor is likely to be true. Human beings have a great capacity to dissemble and to do so quite effectively—that is, without being detected (e.g., Bond & DePaulo, 2006). We might agree with Wilkins if what he meant was that, over long periods of time, therapists cannot consistently offer UPR unless it feels genuine. But all therapists have sometimes "faked it," especially when they have been tested or provoked or worked when they were not at their best. We've all strained to be patient and accepting and caring when patients push past our limits at a given moment or session.

Research conducted by the senior author's research team has shed some light on the extent to which therapists are not always honest in their dealings with clients. In the largest of the studies done on this topic (Jackson et al., 2022), a homogeneous sample of therapists ($N = 401$, mean age = 46.3, mean years of clinical experience = 16.5) was presented with 23 items that reflect instances of possible therapist dishonesty (e.g., "Have you ever given a client the impression that you remembered something when in fact you didn't?"). Results of this study indicated that being dishonest about feelings toward a client is not at all an unusual occurrence. Furthermore, two of the five most highly ranked items concerned (a) therapists' feelings of frustration or disappointment and (b) therapists' feelings of liking a client.

Therapists can and do occasionally fake feelings of PR for their clients. Whether they can do so consistently over long periods of time is a question that has not yet been answered. But, based on these survey results, here is what we do know: 41.4% of therapists surveyed in this study acknowledged that they were at least sometimes (4 on a 7-point scale) dishonest about how much they liked their clients, and 46.9% acknowledged that they were at least sometimes dishonest about their feelings of frustration or disappointment with their clients. Thus, a substantial minority—approaching 50%—of therapists sometimes faked feelings of liking and hid feelings of frustration or disappointment. Moreover, there were no significant differences in this study in respondents' scores on these items as a function of theoretical orientation. Statistically speaking, humanistic therapists were as likely to dissemble as any other type of therapist.

PR, like other strong emotions or attitudes, including love or anger, waxes and wanes in its intensity and authenticity. There may well be some constant, minimal sense of accepting or loving a client, friend, child, or significant other, but all of us are aware that these feelings fluctuate as a function of our mood and needs, others' mood and needs, and some interaction effect. Even when therapists consistently care deeply about a client, the tone and behaviors reflecting their caring and acceptance inevitably shift from session to session and over time. And sometimes, as in a mother's attunement to her baby, one may seem to have all the right moves, but one's heart is not quite in it (Stern, 1985). Rogers (1959) believed this as well, noting that PR occurs in varying degrees at different times. Our sense, then, is that PR can be faked, and effectively so, though it is likely that there are limits to how much this can occur before a client senses the disingenuousness and no longer feels positively regarded.

Are There Both Proximal and Distal Effects of Positive Regard?

Wilkins (2000/2001) proposed that at times, UPR, filtered through acutely attuned empathy, can strike the exact right notes and have an immediate salutary effect on clients. He offered, as an example, a remark he made to a client who was complaining bitterly about a coworker who wasn't pulling his weight:

> As he described all this to me, without really thinking, I said, "You wish he would fuck off and die." There was instantly a look of profound relief on Jim's face and, at first softly and then with increasing vehemence, he repeated my phrase several times. (p. 45)

Wilkins (2000/2001) then imagined how his intervention made a difference: "Somehow the phrase I used seemed to have the right force. . . . In some way he was changed by hearing me acceptingly voice his hidden wish" (p. 45).

Wilkins went on to note that this level of deep reflection, one where the empathic remark offered resonates strongly with a feeling just below the surface level, is an extremely powerful, deeply affecting experience.

Bauman (2001) seemed to be in agreement with this view when he wrote:

> Perhaps the most powerful growthful moment in therapy occurs when the client experiences new clarity of a heretofore unavailable aspect of his/her experience arising from the therapist's communication of empathic understanding, *followed by the client's experience of no reduction in the therapist's need or willingness to know the client*. (p. 3, italics in original)

Bauman (2001) was describing an epiphany, a great sense on the part of the client that "Oh my God, I can be true to myself" and still have my therapist not only accept me but genuinely seek contact with me (p. 4). Wilkins's and Bauman's views, as well as those of Lietaer (2001), are solidly in the realm of a corrective emotional experience (Castonguay & Hill, 2012), a realization of new possibilities brought on by the therapist's acceptance.

These observations here are somewhat in contrast with the usual sense that the effects of PR are gradual, discernible only after repeated efforts made by the therapist to demonstrate that the therapist's care and acceptance are enduring, real, and essentially unconditional. Rogers's extensive therapeutic work (166 sessions) with Jim Brown, a 28-year-old man diagnosed as schizophrenic and displaying symptoms of severe depression, reveals this pattern. In reviewing his treatment of Mr. Brown, Rogers (1967) wrote the following, among the most poignant descriptions of his work across his entire career:

> In this relationship there was a moment of real, and I believe irreversible change. Jim Brown, who sees himself as stubborn, bitter, mistreated, worthless, useless, hopeless, unloved, unlovable, experiences my caring. In that moment, his defensive shell cracks wide open and can never again be quite the same. When someone cares for him, and he feels and experiences that caring, he becomes a softer person whose years of stored-up hurt come pouring out in anguished sobs. He is not the shell of hardness and bitterness, the stranger to tenderness. He is a person hurt beyond words, and aching for the love and caring which alone can make him human. (p. 411)

It is likely, therefore, that the effects of PR can be experienced intensely by clients in the moment, as in Wilkins's example, or more gradually, by degrees, as in Rogers's example preceding. Similarly, other writers (e.g., Farber et al., 2012) have suggested that the corrective emotional experience that results from the therapist's caring can occur as the result of the cumulative impact of a session or sessions or as emanating from moments of intense attunement.

Is Positive Regard an Attitude or a Set of Behaviors?

One of the most difficult questions to answer about PR is how it is actually enacted. Rogers never really answered this question directly, preferring to regard it as an overall attitude encompassing aspects of warmth, caring, respect, interest, and acceptance—aspects that are typically mediated through the therapist's empathy. Sometimes, too, Rogers (1961) would add a more spiritual or transcendent perspective, suggesting that, over time, a therapist's acceptance and respect "tends to change to something approaching awe as he sees the valiant and deep struggle of the person to be himself" (p. 82). Aligning himself somewhat with this latter perspective, Iberg (2001) maintained that the person expressing UPR should use all of their senses to be able to fully appreciate the beauty in another, "attending to the full rich detail" and allowing themselves to be fully moved by the other (p. 124). In a similar vein, Hendricks (2001) described UPR as an interaction within which individuals "participate in a joyful, thick, textured aliveness" (p. 133).

There have been other attempts to more fully flesh out the nature and dimensions of a therapist's positively regarding stance. Brodley and Schneider (2001), for example, attempted to synthesize Rogers's various writings about this idea:

> The qualities communicated are the therapist's consistent acceptant understanding of the client's experienced and communicated internal frame of reference, the therapist's consistency in expression of warm interest in the client, and the therapist's consistent attention to the client's self-representations. . . . This *empathic orientation* to the client means that the therapist understands and is receptive to whatever the client is feeling or however the client is construing experiences. (p. 157)

They contended, too, that UPR is communicated by what is omitted in the therapist's communicative repertoire (Brodley & Schneider, 2001). That is, the absence of judgmental statements and suggestions, interpretations, leading questions, and confrontations provides the clear impression that the therapist is fully accepting of the client.

Imagine, then, a therapist, with a body posture approximating that of Carl Rogers—slight lean forward, eyes directed toward the client with barely any shifting, feet flat on the floor—sitting a bit closer to their client than one might expect; occasionally nodding or offering a relaxed smile to denote that they have heard what is being said; constantly trying to understand and sense what the client is experiencing ("vicarious introspection"; Kohut, 1959); restating a client's narrative to check and clarify its emotional meaning; speaking gently, clearly, directly, and with a constant focus on the client's issues and needs; and remaining patient—resisting any urges to provide suggestions, advice, or interpretations of a client's words—instead steadfastly believing that the client will find a way to best guide their own life.

A persistent struggle in conceptualizing PR lies in the dialectic between offering specific examples of what PR "is" in the moment (e.g., specific words that reflect exquisite examples of empathy, prizing, or acceptance) versus insisting that it is primarily an attitude that cannot be reduced to fragments of a dialogue. Our sense is that it can be both. One can provide examples wherein a well-attuned empathic statement—as in Wilkins's example above—seems to have the effect of making the client feel perfectly understood and accepted, resulting in a clear and sometimes dramatic in-the-moment effect. But, even in this example, there's a context to consider: weeks, or perhaps months or even years, in which the therapist consistently provided Rogers's facilitative conditions, likely setting the stage for the just-right statement that had such an impact. This client had begun to accept the possibility that the way in which he has been consistently treated—accepted, prized, cared about—just might be a valid reflection of who he truly is. He had gradually moved to a position of self-acceptance wherein a single "perfect" sentence from his therapist or moments of a therapeutic dialogue could be intensely meaningful, even corrective.

More typically, though, clinical cases do not contain moments of epiphany. Clinical work proceeds slowly and nonlinearly, yielding small-to-moderate improvements in clients' lives. We offer our clients a genuinely felt appreciation of who they are; we accept them as fully as possible; we prize them as individuals; we feel warmly toward them; we show a genuine interest in understanding their lives, including their struggles and their achievements. Over time, without Hollywood endings, they begin to accept themselves in ways that approximate how we have accepted them. We have more to say about how exactly therapists offer this acceptance—what kinds of statements they make, what kinds of accommodations to clients' clinical needs they make, what kinds of nonverbal behaviors they exhibit, and what kinds of seemingly non-PR behaviors nonetheless are experienced by clients as positively regarding—in later chapters.

Is Unconditional Positive Regard Unbiased, and Must It Be Absolutely Nondirective?

Can a therapist, even one attempting to adhere faithfully to the principles of person-centered therapy, maintain an attitude of UPR? Is it not inevitable that a therapist's own needs, biases, and fears will affect their responsiveness to certain client words or themes more than others? Can a therapist be so nonjudgmental and unconditional such that their gaze, smile, attentiveness, interest, and verbal tone are absolutely unwavering regardless of what the client speaks about? Multiple clinicians, theorists, and researchers have grappled with this issue, with those outside the fold of person-centered therapy—including such luminaries as Rollo May and Albert Ellis—contesting most vehemently the notion that a therapist, especially one with a positive bias toward human nature, could be absolutely nonjudgmental.

One of the first significant challenges to Rogers's contention that a therapist can consistently adopt a nonjudgmental stance was by Charles Truax, a student and later colleague of Rogers and someone with whom Rogers had a documented contentious relationship (Kirschenbaum, 1979; Rogers & Russell, 2002). In 1966, Truax published a now oft-cited article with the provocative title "Reinforcement and Nonreinforcement in Rogerian Psychotherapy." Using a team of clinical judges, Truax analyzed a long-term, seemingly successful psychotherapy case of Rogers, attempting to determine the extent to which Rogers varied his responses, including his warmth and empathy, as a function of specific instances of his client's words and behaviors, or whether, per client-centered tenets, his responses were noncontingent.

Truax's (1966) findings suggested that Rogers responded differentially to several classes of patient behavior. For example, when the patient's style of speech essentially mirrored Rogers's style, Rogers was more empathic, warm, and accepting—and also less directive. Rogers's use of "uh huh" and "mmm mmm" was also reportedly nonrandom: These expressions tended to occur more frequently following client expressions of negative affect. According to Truax, these results showed that Rogers either consciously or unconsciously used empathy, acceptance, and directiveness to selectively reinforce certain client behaviors. Similarly, Truax and Carkhuff (1967), analyzing a greater number of cases, concluded that "client-centered therapists seem less open to receiving negative, hostile or aggressive feelings" than positive feelings (p. 503).

Subsequent research on this issue, however, failed to support these findings. In the most direct rebuttal of this work, and employing a more sophisticated methodological approach, Brodley and Bradburn (2015) examined 25 interviews conducted by Rogers, primarily via transcripts of these cases, finding no indication of any positive bias in his responses to client material reflective of positive, negative, mixed, or neutral affective valence. "He did not respond with positive affect more than his clients did nor did he emphasize their positive leanings by acknowledging them with greater affective intensity that he did their negative feelings" (p. 97).

A variation on the charge that client-centered therapists are biased toward attending to clients' positive feelings is the contention that too many therapists within this tradition have strayed from the classical mandate to be *unconditionally* positively regarding (i.e., to refrain from any temptation to be directive and/or supportive). They have, in the phrase adopted by Freire (2001), assumed that "conditional positive regard" is sufficient (p. 148). For Freire (2001), among others, the therapist's UPR is central to the value of person-centered therapy—its most distinctive feature. From Freire's perspective, any attempt, whether driven by benign motives or the therapist's own narcissism, to move the client in a direction that is not the client's own, is a mistake—a critical violation of a fundamental principle.

These views on the matter of conditionality seem to us rather inflexible. They are far more orthodox than those of Rogers himself, who, as we noted earlier, became more flexible in his approach over time. Moreover, Rogers (1959) was aware of the problematic nature of the word "unconditional" in describing the need for a therapist's PR of clients. He understood that it connoted an all-or-nothing condition and that in or out of psychotherapy, UPR was likely to occur only sometimes—and even then, in varying degrees. In delineating the fundamental conditions of his brand of therapeutic work, he wrote that the therapist's provision of PR needed to be perceived by the client "at least to a minimal degree" (Rogers, 1959, p. 213).

Freire's (2001) examples of conditional PR fall primarily into two categories: therapist attempts to lead sessions and efforts to provide explicit support of clients. According to Freire and others (e.g., Lietaer, 2001), when therapists attempt to lead or direct sessions, they are expressing their lack of faith in the client's ability to direct their own life; the message given is that the client's self-directing capacities are inadequate and not to be trusted. The primary means of falling into this trap is through the therapist's questioning clients in ways that don't reflect the client's narrative at the moment or encouraging clients (even if gently) to go deeper into their current narrative than they have already done. We wonder, though, the following: Whereas Rogers did not offer his own opinion or suggestions about whether Gloria (the client in the demonstration interview) should tell her daughter about her sex life—a position consistent with Freire's and more generally with client-centered doctrine—would Rogers or Freire have maintained this position if Gloria had wondered aloud whether it was a good idea for her to hit or verbally abuse her children? Wouldn't a therapist be well advised to help a parent make a wiser choice if that therapist truly knew what the wiser parenting choice was?

Freire's (2001) second example of conditionality is that of explicit therapist support—an issue, as we've noted previously, that has long been the source of debate within the person-centered movement. In principle, Rogers was opposed to this, contending that any direct indication of a therapist's support for a client's behavior was an imposition, a clear marker of the therapist's values and preferences and not those of the client. Among others, Brodley and Schneider (2001) expressed support for this position, contending that UPR requires that the therapist abjure from either approval or criticism. But on multiple occasions, Rogers himself violated this principle, and others within the person-centered tradition (e.g., Lietaer, 2001) have been liberal in their interpretation of just how inviolable this principle needs to be. In fact, despite the sentiment expressed above by Brodley and Schneider, in a later portion of their paper, they noted that "there may be, of course, exceptions to the therapist's evaluation-neutral presence . . . there are no absolutes in this method" (p. 156). But there are absolutes for Freire. She considers therapist support a technical error, even when it is in the service of helping desperate, confused, or fearful clients: "Whenever the therapist encourages a client, she is not accepting the client's fear. Whenever the therapist enlightens, she is not accepting the client's confusion. Whenever the therapist comforts, she is not accepting the client's desperation" (p. 149).

We don't agree with this assessment. We believe instead that therapists can empathize with a client's fears, confusion, or desperation and utter words of encouragement, clarification, or comfort—and that doing so neither fundamentally undermines nor reflects a disrespect for the client's prerogatives and ability to find their own way through distress. From Freire's perspective, "I can sense how painful this is to you" would be acceptable, but adding, "and I believe you can find your way through it" (i.e., words of support and encouragement) would not be acceptable.

We have more to say about orthodox adherence to the theoretical principles in person-centered therapy when we devote our attention more fully to the controversies and criticisms attendant to the use of PR (see Chapter 9).

Can a Therapist Be Both Rogerian and Eclectic?

There is yet another aspect of nonorthodoxy, that of believing strongly in Rogers's fundamental ideas and seeing oneself as part of the person-centered community but not believing that the core, therapist-provided conditions must be provided within a strict PCA. This is a countervailing perspective to that of Freire's, one that holds that a broad definition and a broad context to the communication of PR are not contaminating influences.

One exemplar of this position is Arthur (Art) Bohart (2015), once a true believer and self-acknowledged "radical person-centered therapist" (p. 1060). Bohart undertook an unusual and unusually thoughtful professional journey, one that led him to becoming an "integrative Rogerian therapist" (p. 1062). He believed in Rogers's fundamental proposition that individuals possess a significant self-actualizing tendency, but Bohart emphasized—even more than Rogers himself—that clients were the active agents of their own growth and healing.

From this realization, Bohart concluded that he could and should legitimately offer clients the "full armamentarium of therapy" (p. 1063), including not only person-centered and existential approaches but also aspects of cognitive behavioral, psychodynamic, and strategic-structural therapies as well. Clients could take of these techniques as they chose or needed, adopting those that were useful and ignoring or discarding those that did not seem helpful.

But there was one more iteration in Bohart's career—essentially, a return to his person-centered roots, a renewed awareness that therapy was fundamentally a deep encounter between two individuals and that techniques were, at best, secondary phenomena. "Therapy is the process of giving clients space and support where they can begin to feel safe" (Bohart, 2015, p. 1066). Although clients might transform some clinical techniques or interventions to meet their own needs, Bohart's (2015) sense was that, fundamentally, therapists need to be sensitive listeners:

> I now say that you can put the whole Rogerian treatment plan in one word, or, if you wrote a Rogerian treatment manual it would consist of one word: Listen. Sensitively responding, offering techniques at timely times, are all forms of being responsive (Stiles, Honos-Webb, & Surko, 1998), of being in dialogue (Schmid, 2004), and therefore are forms of sensitively listening, as is responding with "therapeutic" self-disclosures and "confrontations" if one is coming from an existential point of view. (p. 1066)

In a commentary he wrote in his role as a discussant on a panel about PR at a pandemic-aborted Society for Psychotherapy Research conference, Bohart (2020) further emphasized the extent to which PR, as well as empathy and congruence, needed to be seen not as a one-person (therapist) intervention but rather as part of an interpersonal encounter. PR, he noted, should be seen as a meeting of two persons, in which one person relates to the other with unconditional respect, as if the other person is a person worthy of being respected, appreciated, and listened to; in short, making the other feel as if they truly matter. Here, Bohart's ideas overlap considerably with the practice of contemporary relational psychodynamic practitioners as well as those adopting an attachment-based psychotherapy.

Thus, Bohart now feels free to offer clients aspects of what he's learned about multiple forms of psychotherapy. He believes in sharing the wisdom he's accrued from many sources. As he explained it,

> I have returned to my radical early Rogerian roots, only now with a more balanced perspective. I no longer see it as either/or: either I listen or I use techniques. I do listen. But as a part of listening and relating on a person-to-person basis, I see it as honoring the person to offer whatever thoughts and experiences I have in their service, that they may find useful. (Bohart, 2015, p. 1067)

In short, Bohart demonstrates his respect and PR for his clients not just through acceptance and empathy—the "classical" Rogerian routes—but also through providing whatever wisdom and knowledge are at his disposal. As we ourselves do, we suspect that many therapists admire this position.

Is Therapeutic Presence a Useful Means of Understanding the Essence of Positive Regard?

A therapeutic attitude or stance that bears a good deal of resemblance to Rogers's ideas about PR is *therapeutic presence*, "a way of being that reflects therapists' full engagement in the moment-to-moment encounter with their client" (S. M. Geller, 2013, p. 209) or, in Schneider's (2015) words, "a complex mix of appreciative openness, concerted engagement, support, and expressiveness" (p. 304). This engagement optimally occurs on emotional, cognitive, spiritual, and physical levels. Consistent with Rogers's theories (and Bohart's experience), the achievement of therapeutic presence is said to facilitate clients' innate tendency toward growth.

S. M. Geller's (2013) chapter synthesizing the theory of and research on therapeutic presence was published in *The Handbook of Person-Centred Psychotherapy and Counselling* (Cooper et al., 2013), reflecting the essential place of this relational attitude within the overall world of person-centered psychotherapy. She emphasized the ways in which therapeutic presence provides a safe and supportive connection for clients, concomitantly generating a highly attuned and mutually beneficial therapeutic relationship. She suggested that therapeutic presence is the foundation for Rogers's core conditions—"the preliminary necessity of receptively being clear and open to receive the totality of the client's and one's own experience" (S. M. Geller, 2013, p. 211)—and that Rogers himself implicitly supported this idea. To substantiate this assertion, she cited an interview during which Rogers expressed the thought that "it is something around the edges of those [facilitative] conditions that is really the most important element of therapy—when my self is very clearly, obviously present" (cited in Baldwin, 2000, p. 30). In a similar vein, Schneider (2015) contended that presence is the central, unifying element across those common or contextual factors that exist across all therapeutic orientations and that account for much of therapy's effectiveness.

S. M. Geller and Greenberg (2012) emphasized the specific connection between therapeutic presence and empathy, contending that presence may be a prerequisite for true empathy. They noted, too, preliminary findings confirming the positive association between these variables (S. M. Geller et al., 2010). In a related vein, Watson and Greenberg (2009), adopting a neuroscience perspective and invoking the notion of mirror neurons, suggested the use of the term "empathic resonance" to refer to therapists' attempts to understand clients' experience. To the extent that empathy is often the primary modality by which PR is conveyed, and to the extent that therapists' inability to be fully present is likely to interfere with their capacity to fully understand and accept their clients, therapeutic presence may be one part of a comprehensive understanding of the mechanisms involved in the communication of PR.

To What Extent Does Gendlin's Practice of "Focusing" Overlap With Rogers's Practice of Positive Regard?

Earlier in this chapter, we briefly invoked Gendlin's name in discussing whether a therapist's countertransferential responses—the therapist's articulated feelings about the client and the therapy—could be legitimately placed within the category of PR. Gendlin, we noted, was solidly in this camp, believing that even expressions of anger or frustration, so long as they were expressed in a respectful manner, were indications of an overall caring attitude.

Arguably, Gendlin was the most prominent of neo-Rogerians, a philosopher who studied and collaborated with Rogers at the University of Chicago. He was a coeditor, along with Rogers, Grendlin, Kiesler, and Truax (1967), of a book-length treatment of their work using client-centered therapy with individuals diagnosed with schizophrenia: *The Therapeutic Relationship and Its Impact: A Study of Psychotherapy With Schizophrenics*. Although not a psychologist, Gendlin was the recipient of multiple achievement awards by different divisions of the American Psychological Association and was also the recipient of a lifetime achievement award from the World Association for Person Centered and Experiential Psychotherapy and Counseling.

Gendlin's movement away from, or beyond, classical client-centered thinking essentially consisted of his variation on Rogers's theory regarding individuals' innate actualizing tendency, their movement toward their full creative potential. Gendlin (1978) thought that he intuited something even more basic, more organic. He referred to this as "bodily knowing," "bodily awareness," or the inner "felt sense" of ongoing life processes. "A felt sense is the wholistic [*sic*], implicit, body sense of a complex situation" (p. 58). He worked with clients to recognize their inner sense of an experience. Moving clients to better recognize their felt lived experience was what Gendlin named "focusing." The therapist's "experiential response" was in the service of helping clients become more acutely aware of their felt experience. An example was offered in Gendlin's (1996) book, *Focusing-Oriented Psychotherapy: A Manual of the*

Experiential Method. Here, he was working with a client who was struggling with a wish to give up smoking marijuana:

CLIENT: It's very interesting, the fear is right underneath it. Now I'm content to sit there with the withdrawn, and feel apathy until I . . . end up with the feeling, then I withdraw into the nice apathy again (*laughs*).

THERAPIST: Mmm, the apathy is more comfortable and the fear is right under it, so you just push down and ah . . . there it is. (*Silence*)

THERAPIST: Well, let's be friendly with the fear, and sort of say, that's all right, right now we're not doing anything. We'd just like to hear from it. What it's so scared about. (p. 31)

We can see that the therapist's first response here was quite Rogerian. Indeed, according to many commentators, person-centered therapy and Gendlin's focusing have much in common. In each model, noted Jaison (2008), therapists strive to be "affirming, listening, and assisting clients in drawing upon what is already intuitively and instinctively known . . . each model emphasizes a way of being with clients that is respectful, non-judgmental, caring" (p. 55).

Whereas this comparison suggests that a clinician operating from Gendlin's model is as positively regarding as one whose treatment is more informed by Rogerian principles, from a strict theoretical perspective, this is not the case. From a classical person-centered view, Gendlin was not as accepting as Rogers. The latter allowed the client to "go" wherever he or she wanted—to speak or not speak, to access emotional content or not, to get to the felt sense of the matter or not. By contrast, Gendlin's brand of therapy has an agenda, one that has much in common with present-day emotion-focused therapy. Clients are encouraged to get to a certain place, a deeply felt, "authentic" experiential place that in Gendlin's view was mutative. Gendlin, then, may well have been supportive, caring, and affirming—all aspects of being positively regarding—but his focusing training does not include another essential aspect of PR, that of being accepting of a client's experience or direction. As Raskin (1987) noted: "Each of the neo-Rogerian methods takes something away from the thorough-going belief in the self-directive capacities that is so central to client-centered philosophy" (p. 460).

In sum, many attempts have been made to reconceptualize Rogers's ideas about UPR as well as his ideas about PR writ large. Not surprisingly, many of these newer conceptualizations have been made with considerable pushback from those adhering to traditional client-centered perspectives. Although we are sympathetic to the view that therapist acceptance of clients—their needs, indeed, their basic personhood—is an inviolable principle, we are far more ardent supporters of the general proposition that there are multiple means of adopting an overall positively regarding attitude toward clients. We believe that absolute, nonjudgmental acceptance, per the dictates of the classical Rogerian position, is one avenue toward this overall goal—but we also believe that there are other pathways, encompassing ideas and techniques from other theoretical perspectives, that are equally capable of demonstrating a caring, affirming, and highly respectful attitude toward clients. We develop these ideas further in subsequent chapters.

4 PR-LIKE CONCEPTS OUTSIDE THE PERSON-CENTERED COMMUNITY

Some come dark and strange like dying/crows and ravens whistling
Lines of weeping, strings of crying/so much said in listening

—Joni Mitchell, "Songs to Aging Children Come"

As we noted in the previous chapter, multiple theorists within the person-centered approach (PCA) community have proposed modifications to various aspects of Carl Rogers's ideas about positive regard (PR). But, for the most part, they adopted the same nomenclature and refrained from reformulating its basic tenets. By contrast, several theorists unaligned with the person-centered world have promulgated concepts that, while overlapping considerably with Rogerian ideas about PR, reflect significant variations in form and name. Some, like Irvin Yalom, are part of a larger constellation of humanistic-existential therapists; others, like Donald Winnicott (object relations), John Bowlby (attachment theory), Heinz Kohut (self psychology), Stephen Mitchell and Paul Wachtel (relational dynamic psychotherapy), Aaron and Judith Beck (cognitive therapy), and William Miller (motivational interviewing), are distinctly aligned with other therapeutic traditions; and still others, such as Marsha

https://doi.org/10.1037/0000312-005
Understanding and Enhancing Positive Regard in Psychotherapy: Carl Rogers and Beyond,
by B. A. Farber, J. Y. Suzuki, and D. Ort

Linehan (dialectical behavior therapy [DBT]), have adopted a more eclectic approach to the practice of psychotherapy. We have selected these diverse clinical approaches as evidence of the manner in which a remarkable range of theoretical traditions have generated their own takes on PR.

In this chapter, we review how these theorists have utilized aspects of the PR concept within their own work, how their understanding of this attitude compares to that of Rogers, and the ways in which contemporary therapists of all types might incorporate these ideas into their own practice. In noting points of commonality with Rogers's conception of PR, we aim to highlight PR as a transtheoretical construct that has near-universal significance for the practice of psychotherapy as a whole. At the same time, an appreciation of the differences between these approaches and person-centered therapy can offer clinicians across multiple perspectives a deeper understanding of those aspects of PR that may underlie and vitalize their work, allowing them to select and contextualize expressions of PR within their chosen orientation.

IRVIN YALOM AND "NEED-FREE LOVE"

Irvin Yalom is a self-described American existential psychiatrist who, in addition to writing several influential texts for the field (e.g., *Existential Psychotherapy*, 1980; *The Theory and Practice of Group Psychotherapy*, 1995), has also published several compilations of case material (e.g., *Momma and the Meaning of Life: Tales of Psychotherapy*, 2020; *Love's Executioner and Other Tales of Psychotherapy*, 2012), a heartfelt "letter" to burgeoning psychotherapists (*The Gift of Therapy: An Open Letter to a New Generation of Therapists and Their Patients*, 2002), and several best-selling novels in which psychotherapy is a prominent theme (e.g., *When Nietzsche Wept*, 1992; *The Schopenhauer Cure: A Novel*, 2005). He has been a prolific and "must-read" author for several generations of therapists across multiple theoretical orientations. Through his books and videos, he has modeled an existential therapy that, in addition to emphasizing the importance of considering the "ultimate concerns" of death, isolation, freedom, and meaninglessness, has highlighted the importance of an authentic client–therapist relationship.

Yalom's case material reveals a therapist who has adopted much of Rogers's style—he is consistently empathic, open, warm, valuing, and caring and places great emphasis on the "here and now" of therapy and the mutative power inherent in an egalitarian therapeutic relationship. "Therapy," Yalom (2002) suggested, "should not be theory-driven but relationship driven" (p. xv).

Moreover, Yalom's relationship with his clients shares much in common with Rogers's (1961) description of a therapist's PR:

> His attitude, at its best, is devoid of the quid pro quo aspect of most of the experiences we call love. It is the simple outgoing human feeling of one individual for another, a feeling, it seems to me which is even more basic than sexual or parental feeling. It is a caring enough about the person that you do not wish to interfere with his development, not to use him for any self-aggrandizing goals of your own. Your satisfaction comes in having set him free to grow in his own fashion. (p. 84)

Yalom's (1980) preferred terms for these qualities include "need-free" love and "therapeutic eros" (p. 364). Moreover, wrote Yalom, therapists should not direct their clients but rather help them find their own unique self: "The therapist's raison d'être is to be midwife to the birth of the patient's yet unlived life" (p. 408).

So what, then, are the differences? Is Yalom a de facto Rogerian in the ways in which he provides PR toward his clients? In fact, no. There are similarities, to be sure, in the ways in which they are exquisitely attuned to and affirming of their clients. However, there are at least three fundamental differences in their approach to clients.

One fundamental difference concerns Rogers's imperative that therapists should be both unconditionally accepting and nondirective. Yalom, unlike Rogers but consistent with an existential approach to therapy, moves clients toward confronting their ultimate concerns. An example of this can be seen in Yalom's (2012) work with a client in *Love's Executioner and Other Tales of Psychotherapy*: In the beginning of their therapeutic encounter, Yalom recounted

> again and again [inviting] Marvin to look within, to adopt, even for a moment, a cosmic perspective, to identify the deeper concerns of his existence—his sense of finitude, of aging and decline, his fear of death, his source of life purpose. But we talked past each other. He ignored me, misunderstood me. (p. 241)

Although Yalom is careful, in a very Rogerian manner, to check his understanding of what the client is saying and ask if his interpretations "sound right," he is the guide. He is the person who, if not having the answers, at least suggests the roadmap to search for these answers. In Marvin's case, as the course of therapy continues, Yalom's (2012) guidance ultimately leads Marvin to the point where he has to decide "how to face the pitiless existential facts of life: death, isolation, groundlessness, and meaninglessness" (p. 267). Yalom may well do this in the most caring, accepting way, but he has a sense as to where his clients should go to become more fully self-actualized. Rogers, of course, does not. And yet, one senses that the existential therapist's insistence on confronting these ultimate concerns is grounded in a deep sense of respect analogous to that of the person-centered therapist. Where the former might say, "I respect you too much to tell you what to think," the latter might counter, "I respect you too much to allow the true meaning of your life to pass you by."

A second distinction concerns the limits and value of therapist disclosure, specifically as it implicates the therapist's PR. Yalom's (2002) work features an almost unfettered tendency to self-disclose: "I never let an hour go by without checking into our relationship, sometimes with a simple statement like: 'How are you and I doing today?' or 'How are you experiencing the space between us today?'" (p. 12). Yalom's work is consistent with the position that, communicated genuinely and caringly, disclosures of even negative feelings and consistent reflections about the relationship can not only strengthen trust within the dyad but may also serve as powerful provisions of PR. Rogers, while extolling the virtues of genuineness, was far more conservative in this regard.

The extent of self-disclosure Yalom exhibits within his case material is often quite remarkable. He allows his clients—and his readers—to see him as quite vulnerable. His self-disclosures are at times unflattering. Perhaps the most striking instance of this is Yalom's (2012) candid disclosure of his own prejudice against overweight women, exemplified in his work with his client Betty. When approaching termination due to Betty's upcoming move, Yalom reassures her that she will have the ability to trust others and reveal herself again the way she has in their therapy. But he also acknowledges a difficult and shameful truth:

> I'll miss our meetings. But I'm changed as a result of knowing you. . . . What I mean is that my attitude about obesity has changed a lot. When we started I personally didn't feel comfortable with obese people—In unusually feisty terms, Betty interrupted me. "Ho! ho! ho! 'Didn't feel comfortable'—that's putting it mildly. Do you know that for the first six months you hardly ever looked at me? And in a whole year and a half you've never—not once—touched me? Not even for a handshake!" My heart sank. My God, she's right! I have never touched her. I simply hadn't realized it. And I guess I didn't look at her very often, either. I hadn't expected her to notice! . . . I saw I had no choice but to own up. (pp. 137–138)

The two then candidly and warmly discuss how Betty had experienced the therapeutic relationship, and Yalom is open to criticism from, and willing to be instructed by, his client. This interaction ultimately leads to an even deeper and more amicable parting that seems to convey sincere and genuine—if imperfect—respect. In his willingness to have these hard conversations, disclose his own biases and shortcomings, and work on the relationship with his clients, Yalom exhibits what might be considered an extended form of Rogers's PR by trusting his clients with his own vulnerability and prejudice.

The third distinction may well be the most critical. Unlike Rogers, Yalom unequivocally advocates for actively affirming clients, including offering them compliments for who they are and what they've done; as such, he models a significant expansion of the concept of PR beyond what Rogers proposed. Yalom believes that therapists should, as often as possible, celebrate clients' abilities to adapt, change, or grow. He highlights the fact that there is an authority afforded therapists by their clients. Clients generally trust their therapists, share their most intimate selves, and value their therapists' opinions and perceptions. Actively affirming and even celebrating clients verbally provides them with evidence that whatever maladaptive beliefs they have about themselves cannot be entirely accurate, as their respected therapist thinks otherwise. What is it, Yalom (2002) asked, that clients remember about their therapeutic experiences?

> Not insight nor the therapist's interpretations. More often than not, they remember the positive supportive statements of their therapist. I make a point of regularly expressing my positive thoughts and feelings about my patients, along a wide range of attributes—for example, their social skills, intellectual curiosity, warmth, loyalty to their friends, articulateness, courage in facing their inner demons, dedication to change, willingness to self-disclose, loving gentleness with their children, commitment to breaking the cycle of abuse and decision not to pass on the "hot potato" to the next generation. Don't be stingy—there's no point to it; there is every reason to express these observations and your positive sentiments . . . acceptance and support from one who knows you so intimately is enormously affirming. (pp. 423–425)

Here, then, we have an example of a renowned therapist who is avowedly positively regarding toward his clients but in ways that deviate significantly from the original ideas of Rogers and traditional person-centered therapists. Even as Yalom privileges authenticity over classical Rogerian notions of unconditional positive regard (UPR) and eschews nondirectivity almost entirely, he nonetheless relies on a foundation of PR that resonates strongly with the broader, more ecumenical definition of PR allowed by some of Rogers's descendants as described in the previous chapter (e.g., Bohart, 2015; Lietaer, 2001; Wilkins, 2000/2001). Thus, Yalom's work offers one rich example of how a therapist's broadly constituted regard for clients, expressed sincerely and incorporated effectively into a distinct clinical theory, can have a catalyzing effect on their shared healing journeys.

D. W. WINNICOTT AND THE HOLDING ENVIRONMENT

Donald (D. W.) Winnicott (1896–1971) was a seminal figure in the development and clinical applications of object relations theory, a psychoanalytic movement that rejected Freud's notions of the motivational significance of drives (sex and aggression), positing instead that early interpersonal relationships were the essential determinants of personality and psychopathology. Winnicott and other object relations theorists set the stage for the emergence, in the late 20th century, of relational psychodynamic psychotherapy.

Winnicott began his career as a pediatrician, a role that shaped much of his clinical theorizing. Drawing upon his extensive experience with mothers and babies, he conceptualized the idea of the "good enough mother." It was, he thought, the mother's responsiveness to the baby's needs and the quality of the environment she provides—a "holding environment"—that shapes the individual's sense of self. "We are more concerned," Winnicott (1955) wrote, "with the mother *holding* the baby than with the mother *feeding* the baby" (p. 148)—a statement entirely consistent with the work of two of Winnicott's contemporaries, John Bowlby (with displaced and hospitalized children) and Harry Harlow (with primates). Further, Winnicott (1960) suggested, this physical and emotional holding must be responsive to the specific needs of a specific baby at a specific time: Holding needs to be "reliable in a way that implies the mother's empathy" (p. 48); it cannot be "mechanical." And in a statement that sounds as if it could have come directly from the writings of Rogers, Winnicott (1990) contended that "in an environment that holds the baby well enough, the baby is able to make personal development according to inherited tendencies" (p. 28).

Winnicott took this notion of a holding environment, one in which the mother is attuned and attentive to the baby's changing needs, and extrapolated it to the psychotherapeutic setting. The therapist provides a holding environment by being reliable (i.e., by having clear boundaries about the nature and "rules" of psychotherapy), empathic, and responsive. The overlaps between the clinical theories of Rogers and Winnicott, and the specific convergence around a core idea resembling UPR, become especially apparent in Modell's (1976) description of the psychotherapist's adherence to Winnicott's ideas about a holding environment:

> The analyst is constant and reliable; he responds to the patient's affects; he accepts the patient, and his judgment is less critical and more benign; he is there primarily for the patient's needs and not for his own; he does not retaliate; and he does at times have a better grasp of the patient's inner psychic reality than does the patient himself and therefore may clarify what is bewildering and confusing. (p. 291)

The parallels to Roger's concept of nonpossessive warmth here are striking. Except for the last sentence suggesting that the therapist has a better grasp of the patient's "psychic reality" than the patient themself—a sentiment antithetical to Rogers's beliefs—these attributes are quite consistent with Rogers's insistence on the need for therapists to be accepting, benign, and attuned to the affective tone of the client's narrative. Moreover, in this quotation, Modell may be misrepresenting Winnicott's beliefs regarding "who knows best." Whereas Winnicott did not eliminate interpretation from his repertoire—as a psychoanalyst, he believed in its usefulness—Winnicott's (1969) description of his use of this technique reflects a client-centered sensibility: "I think I interpret mainly to let the patient know the limits of my understanding. The principle is that it is the patient and only the patient who has the answers" (p. 711). Again, the spirit underlying this statement, if not its precise technical meaning, powerfully evokes a Rogerian sensibility.

S. A. Mitchell and Black's (1995) understanding of Winnicott's holding environment provides further evidence of the overlap between the ideas of this object relations therapist and that of the founder of client-centered therapy:

> The analyst, like the good enough mother, tries to grasp the deeply personal dimensions of the patient's experience, the patient's spontaneously arising desires. The patient is offered refuge from the demands of the outside world; nothing is expected except to "be" in the analytic situation, to connect with and express what one is experiencing. (p. 133)

The points to be emphasized here are, first, the need for the analyst to be empathic, to grasp the patient's subjectivity and, second, the imperative for the analyst to be absolutely accepting of whatever the patient brings to the therapeutic situation. Winnicott's statement to a patient at the end of an early clinical session reflects both of these dimensions: "I've nothing particular to say yet, but if I don't say something, you may begin to feel I'm not here" (Guntrip, 1996, p. 749). Although Rogers would not have been this interpretive, Winnicott's comments here suggest a Rogerian-like deep empathy and deep caring for his patient.

Both Winnicott and Rogers believed that the therapist's caring—in Winnicott's terms, the provision of a holding environment, and in Rogers's terms, the provision of PR—could substantially undo the psychic damage caused by inadequate parenting. In Winnicott's terms, this damage was attributable to the absence of a good enough mother (parent) who could provide an empathic holding environment; in Rogers's terms, this damage was attributable to conditions of worth (i.e., parents' communication to children that they are lovable only if they adhere to parental dictates and values). Thus, while the tenets of object relations theory and person-centered theory differ significantly in their focus and metapsychologies, they nonetheless have undeniable commonalities as expressed in the treatment room, converging primarily around attitudes of empathic understanding and warm acceptance (whether termed a "holding environment" or "unconditional positive regard") that their founders agreed were central mechanisms of change in the therapeutic process.

JOHN BOWLBY, MARY AINSWORTH, AND CLIENTS' NEED FOR A SECURE BASE

In developing attachment theory, John Bowlby (along with his too-often overlooked collaborator, Mary Ainsworth) contended that a healthy, secure attachment between mother and child was predicated on the mom's consistent responsiveness to the child's needs. Mother (or other caretaker) needed to provide "a warm, intimate, and continuous relationship . . . in which both find satisfaction and enjoyment" in order to facilitate the growth of a "mentally healthy" individual who could experience a basic sense of trust in the world (Bowlby, 1951, p. 11).

Bowlby dedicated the last 10 years or so of his professional life to transposing the principles underlying attachment theory to psychotherapeutic practice. In adopting an attachment-based clinical model, therapists are enjoined to provide their clients a secure base, recapitulating to a great extent the conditions in childhood that facilitate secure attachments. It is the therapist's constancy, availability, sensitivity, and responsiveness that catalyze the establishment of a secure base; therapists working within this model strive to be predictably responsive to the needs of their clients, attuning to their affective world and attending to both verbal and nonverbal material (Farber et al., 1995; Farber & Metzger, 2009). According to Bowlby (1977, 1988), working in this manner may mean providing comfort, empathy, and understanding; at other times, generating new solutions to problems; and, at still other times, offering explicit encouragement, advice, and guidance. Bowlby contended that if the therapist is able to enact these goals and attitudes, the patient may be able to rework maladaptive attachment patterns and internalize a new "secure base" script, one that facilitates honest client disclosure and allows for client insight into previous relationship patterns and their effect on current relationships.

For the most part, these goals and therapist behaviors resemble greatly those that Rogers touted as essential and specifically with Rogers's notion of PR. Indeed, given that Bowlby positioned attachment theory as a variant of object relations theory and acknowledged that the concept of secure base overlaps considerably with Winnicott's (1965) ideas about a psychologically protective holding environment, it follows that the secure base concept has much in common with Rogers's notion of PR, as well. Leiper and Casares (2000) suggested that "to provide a secure base for the client, the therapist must be perceived to be real, genuine, concerned and in touch with the patient's feelings" (p. 452). However, like other forms of relationally oriented psychodynamic therapy, attachment-based psychotherapy shares features with person-centered therapy but is also distinctive, especially in its imperative for therapists to interpret the meaning and import of past relational events.

The partial transcript that follows is not from Bowlby himself but from Susan Johnson (2009), who adopted an attachment-based model for emotionally focused therapy (EFT) with a client who had symptoms of posttraumatic stress disorder and a fearful-avoidant attachment style. The client, a woman in her 40s, was, in this (10th) session, bemoaning the fact that people, including her mom, forgot about her birthday and that she needed to stop working at a job that provided meaning and satisfaction. The therapist empathized: "Hard to have people miss your birthday, hard to have lost the sense of running that huge machine. That was important to you, wasn't it?" And then:

LESLIE: I was good at running that machine. And at night in that place, it was me that was running it. I knew how to run it. It was my kingdom, and no one else was there.

THERAPIST: Yes. You mattered. You knew how to run the big machine well. You felt strong, confident, and safe there. But you made the choice. You knew that that aloneness and that life was killing you. It was safe but deadly, no?

LESLIE: My cat is the only good thing in my life, No one loves me like her, so I get scared if she looks sick. I just don't trust people.

THERAPIST: Yes. And you have good reasons for that. It's amazing that you have the courage to come here and risk talking about all these things with me.

LESLIE: You challenge me sometimes, but you don't scare me.

THERAPIST: But other people do, don't they, Leslie? They really scare you. There isn't much room for trust, or even giving people a chance. Did you tell people it was your birthday?

LESLIE: (*Looks away.*)
Later, the therapist remarks, "You decide it's safer to be alone, but the longing is still there, isn't it?" and Leslie begins to cry. (Johnson, 2009, pp. 424–425)

The use of PR in this attachment-based therapy is evident: The therapist was empathic ("Hard to have people miss your birthday," "You decide it's safer to be alone, but the longing is still there") and affirming ("Yes. You mattered") and provided Leslie with praise for her courage in seeking help. Still, this therapist also worked to connect what the client was currently saying to things she had said in the past and was far more interpretive and directive (e.g., "But other people . . . really scare you") than a person-centered therapist would be. She attempted to understand (and reflect back to the client) the nature and current manifestations of this client's patterns of relating to others. As Farber and Metzger (2009) noted,

> The concept of secure base provides the ground for therapist-client discussions of what is and "should be" happening between them. "Why, and in what ways," a therapist might well ask, "do I still feel unsafe to you?" "What is it that you keep expecting me to do that keeps us at a distance?" And, "What is it you need from me to feel more connected/more disclosing/more hopeful?" . . . The uniqueness of the secure base concept, then, lies not in its essential features (inasmuch as these have been valued by one or another therapeutic system for many decades) but rather in what its use can lead to: in-depth exploration of the self-in-relationship-to-others. (pp. 50–51)

As with many other therapies, there is an element of PR here as part of the therapist's efforts to empathize with the client, affirm the client's strengths, and fortify the therapeutic relationship. Attachment-based therapies do have a particular aim in mind in offering a secure base—building insight into maladaptive internal working models derived from early attachment relationships—and are thus inherently more directed and directive than most PCA models. From another vantage point, though, the two therapies' provision of something resembling PR aims to accomplish something quite similar: facilitating the client's ability to think, feel, and behave in new, more adaptive, self-congruent ways.

HEINZ KOHUT AND SELF PSYCHOLOGY: EVERYONE NEEDS MIRRORING

In the late 1970s, Heinz Kohut pioneered a new way of understanding and treating patients that would become known as *self psychology*. Much as Rogers decided a quarter of a century earlier, Kohut believed that classical psychoanalytic therapy failed to provide the kind of empathic and affirming experiences necessary for helping patients thrive. Although Kohut broke with psychoanalytic tradition, self psychology has since become highly influential among contemporary psychodynamic theorists, helping to shift psychoanalytic theory and practice closer to Rogers's person-oriented style of therapy.

Kohut did not directly acknowledge Rogers as an influence, even though Rogers's work on empathy was published earlier than Kohut's (Kariagina, 2017; Tobin, 1991). Kohut (1977) noted only that some commentators (e.g., Stolorow, 1976) had remarked on his similarities to other theorists, including Rogers. For his part, Rogers (1987) recognized Kohut as "a major investigator in psychoanalysis" and commented on the similarities and differences between his own work and that of Kohut's; he did so, he stated, mainly as a response to the "often misunderstood" components of the client-centered approach (p. 179).

Much of why Kohut's approach appears to resemble that of Rogers can be traced to similarities in their notions of human development. Broadly speaking, both Rogers and Kohut believed that, given the right environmental conditions, individuals will display a natural tendency toward healthy growth and fulfillment. For Rogers, a healthy environment involves having parents who do not impose conditions of worth on the child. Similarly, for Kohut, healthy development results from the child having had appropriately nurturing experiences with "selfobjects"—Kohut's term for caregivers or, more generally, those persons who serve to affirm individuals' healthy narcissistic needs to experience self-worth and who lead to strengthening the sense of self. Kohut (1971) contended that the root of most psychopathology lies in parental failure to empathize with their children.

Since both Rogers and Kohut assumed that psychopathology is the result of insufficiently nurturing or affirming experiences with others, a crucial role of the therapist, for both theorists, is to provide supportive conditions that allow individuals to pursue their natural tendencies toward growth. For Rogers, this meant that the therapist would be positively regarding, empathic, genuine, and nondirective: The client should lead, and the therapist should avoid all interpretation or goal setting. Kohut (1971, 1977) also believed in the healing power of empathy and of nondirectivity; he contended that simply exposing patients to healthy (essentially affirming) transference experiences with a selfobject—in this case, the therapist—would lead to growth. In some ways, Kohut went further than Rogers in specifying the kinds of affirmation—in Rogers's terms, positive regard—clients need from others in order to restore their wholeness. Kohut posited three types of transferences that could ameliorate clients' unmet early needs: a mirroring transference in which the affirming responses of the therapist begin to allow clients to experience their own worth, an idealizing transference in which the therapist's calm and soothing nature allows clients to feel held and contained, and a twinship transference in which clients begin to identify and mimic the behavior of their therapist. A prominent follower and interpreter of self psychology, Robert Stolorow (1976), proposed a link between Rogers's PR and Kohut's therapeutic attitude as follows:

> The [client-centered] therapist is enjoined to reflect the patient's experiences with an attitude of unconditional positive regard and acceptance, with an eye toward affirming the client's worth, significance and value to the therapist. The client thus comes to experience himself as "prized" by the therapist, much as does the narcissistically disturbed patient immersed in a mirror transference. (p. 28)

Thus, Kohut's self psychology has much in common with the nonjudgmental, accepting, and empathetic attitude encompassed by Rogers's notion of PR. Kohut (1977) suggested that classical psychoanalytic methods involving "lack of emotional responsiveness, silence, the pretense of being an inhuman computer-like machine which gathers data and emits interpretations" are unhelpful and even harmful: "Man can no more survive psychologically in a psychological milieu [i.e., the therapeutic environment] that does not respond empathetically to him than he can survive physically in an atmosphere that contains no oxygen" (p. 253).

However, even though Rogers and Kohut shared somewhat similar thoughts regarding the therapeutic need for a kind of empathy that borders on PR, they diverged in their sense of the place of this attitude within clinical work. Kohut (1977), for his part, suggested that "even the most sensitively responsive behavior from the side of the analyst . . . cannot replace the reconstructive-interpretive approach based upon the analyst's conscious grasp of the patient's structural defects in the self" (p. 259). In other words, Kohut was still working primarily within an analytic frame; interpreting the transference and the patient's past are still primary roles for the self psychologist, even if providing a warm, responsive attitude is both context for interpretations and somewhat helpful independent of interpretations. On the other hand, Rogers (1987) suggested that "when the therapist's understanding is accurate and his acceptance is genuine, when there are no interpretations given and no evaluations made, 'transference' attitudes tend to dissolve, and the feelings are directed toward their true object" (pp. 186–187). One bottom line, though: Kohut and subsequent psychodynamic therapists (see the following) have shown conclusively that clinicians within this tradition can productively incorporate significant aspects of PR into their treatment.

STEPHEN MITCHELL, PAUL WACHTEL, RELATIONAL PSYCHOTHERAPY, AND THE CONCEPT OF "SUPPORT"

Carl Rogers developed his approach to psychotherapy largely in reaction to the hierarchical nature and oft-distant clinical style of psychoanalytic practitioners in the years following World War II. Decades later, relational psychotherapy—arguably the most influential movement within contemporary psychoanalytic thought—would, in turn, embrace what is perhaps the greatest contribution of Rogers to the field: namely, the notion that a supportive therapeutic relationship is critical for success in psychotherapy. Indeed, while relational theories trace their lineage from the interpersonal and object relations traditions within psychoanalysis, rarely crediting their ideas to Rogers himself (Farber, 2007), there is nevertheless a "significant degree of convergence" between Rogers's client-centered view and the tradition of relational psychoanalysis, centering on the notion that "the ground of any effective therapy is a *relationship*" (Wachtel, 2007, p. 280). The findings of a study by Curtis et al. (2004) add credence to the notion of an overlap between contemporary psychoanalytic approaches and person-centered therapy. Surveying analysts about their own analyses, the authors found that among the top 10 interventions viewed by respondents as helpful, there were four that were manifestly Rogerian in nature: the therapist's nonjudgmental and noncritical stance, the therapist's acceptance, the therapist's warmth, and the therapist's validation of one's experiences.

There are, however, important distinctions between person-centered and contemporary (relational) psychodynamic approaches to therapy. These stem largely from the explicit attention given by relational theorists to the role of interpretation and also to conflict and therapeutic ruptures in therapy. Remaining vigilant to the therapeutic potential of recognizing patients' intrapsychic conflicts and therapist–patient conflicts, as virtually all psychoanalytic perspectives tend to do, complicates what the provision of a supportive therapeutic relationship and, in particular, the provision of PR can mean.

Although relational theory rarely mentions Rogers or positive regard per se—Stephen Mitchell's (2000) book *Relationality: From Attachment to Intersubjectivity* somehow neglects to mention Rogers whatsoever—relational theorists frequently engage in tacit channeling of Rogers through discussions of the importance of "support" in therapy, a term that generally refers to therapists' empathic understanding, affirmation, and/or acceptance of patients. Wachtel (2011), much like Kohut before him, summed up the relational perspective's approach to support by writing that

> empathetic immersion in the patient's experience is, I believe, a crucial requirement for therapeutic progress . . . [but] *it is not sufficient.* The view that once true understanding is achieved, everything else takes care of itself oversimplifies and short-circuits the therapeutic process. (p. 192)

Instead, relational theory suggests that within the context of support, therapists must direct their clients toward change through questions, challenges, and interpretations that, in turn, lead to client exploration, insight, and the adoption of new, more adaptive narratives about self and others. Rogers rejected the need for interpretation altogether in favor of a primarily supportive approach. But relational theory, according to Wachtel (2007), holds that "being supportive and being exploratory or depth-oriented are not alternatives but complementary, two sides of a single process . . . [support] entails the provision of the necessary relational nutriment to make genuine insight possible" (p. 169). Furthermore, Wachtel (2007) suggested that helping clients achieve insight into previously unacknowledged aspects of their personalities is precisely how true empathy is communicated:

> The only way to be truly supportive and affirmative . . . is to provide the patient with the experience of being fully understood, or having what at least *he* experiences as the dark side or the weak side acknowledged and known. (p. 162)

In fact, as we see in Chapter 6, this volume, patients in various types of psychotherapy tend to provide implicit support for this view. When asked to evaluate the extent to which a variety of possible actions and statements of their therapist provided them with their sense of being affirmed or positively regarded, the single most highly rated item was "My therapist offers me a new way of understanding a part of myself that I usually view as a weakness" (Suzuki & Farber, 2016).

Summarizing multiple relational perspectives, Wachtel (2007) suggested that the therapist's ability to "not overlook what is uncomfortable" is an essential aspect of true acceptance of the patient. He wrote:

> This is close to what I understand Rogers's (1957) concept of unconditional positive regard to be—not an approval of everything the person does, however insensitive, immoral, or aggressive it might be, but an acceptance of the person as he is, a readiness to view him clearly and wholly and, to the degree possible, to see things through his eyes. (p. 209)

For Wachtel and most relational therapists, acknowledging feelings of hate, or dislike of a client's behavior, does not detract from—and may often even enhance—a therapist's ability to convey true acceptance and PR. Wachtel (2007) succinctly described the effective therapist's stance as "one of striving for unconditional positive regard and inevitably failing in some respects and, therefore, as being confronted with the question of how to be genuine about that failure while still being therapeutic" (p. 281).

Rogers, in recordings and transcripts made of his sessions, was by all appearances so consistently supportive and accepting that one wonders if he was always entirely genuine about his feelings. What of the moments of frustration that relational theorists insist are inevitable? For his part, Rogers did claim, later in his career, "If I am angry, I will express that anger as something within myself, not as a judgment on the other person" (Rogers & Hart, 1970, p. 519). But if, by and large, Rogers's clinical sessions appear to be so consistently devoid of conflict, this may have something to do with his theoretical stance: It is likely easier for a therapist to be more positively regarding, more fully accepting of clients, if the therapy is purposefully nondirective. The relational perspective, by contrast, argues that it is incumbent on therapists to directly call a patient's attention to what needs changing, a mandate that leaves therapists to appear less warm and/or more confrontational. From the perspective of this theoretical orientation, however, this is a trade-off well worth making: If a therapist chooses not to push for deep exploration of the "thoughts and feelings the patient finds most frightening and shameful," Wachtel (2008) noted, "support or affirmation is likely to feel hollow to the patient" (p. 162).

Wachtel (2011) illustrated the relational approach to PR through the case of Frederick, a patient who frequently arrived late to sessions, would miss sessions without notifying the therapist, and hadn't paid his clinic bill in the 5 months since he began therapy. As much as the therapist liked Frederick, his behavior was jeopardizing their relationship and disrupting the treatment. In supervision, Wachtel suggested that rather than challenge Frederick about his behavior, the therapist should communicate acceptance of Frederick's motivations for arriving late and missing sessions, while also suggesting possibilities for change. Frederick's life experiences thus far, which included abandonment, forced migration, and abuse, had left him feeling powerless over his circumstances. Wachtel proposed that the therapist communicate to Frederick his understanding of how important it was for Frederick to regain some sense of power over his life and that arriving late or not paying for sessions could be Frederick's way of saying that, for once, he wanted to do things his way— an attitude that could be chalked up to Frederick's admirable "fighting spirit" (p. 202). At the same time, Wachtel suggested that the therapist should ask Frederick to consider whether there weren't better, less costly ways to gain such a sense of efficacy in his life.

Such an approach is, in a Rogerian sense, positively regarding in that it provides Frederick with conditions of acceptance and even affirmation; but it is also relational in that the therapist focuses on potential conflict within the therapy dyad as a way of identifying what is less acceptable about Frederick's behavior and then nudging him toward change. Despite their differences, it is clear that Rogerian and relational psychotherapies both understand that a supportive therapeutic environment is crucial for providing, as Rogers wrote in 1951, "a safe opportunity for you to discern yourself more clearly, to experience yourself more truly and deeply, to choose more significantly" (p. 35).

CBT THEORISTS AND PRACTITIONERS: TECHNIQUE AND RELATIONAL FACTORS INEVITABLY INTERACT

Marvin Goldfried, one of the most influential researchers and theorists in the behavior therapy and cognitive behavior therapy (CBT) movements, believes that we make a fundamental error in distinguishing between the effects of a therapeutic technique and those emanating from relational factors. They are, he contended (Goldfried & Davila, 2005), inevitably interactive, combining to produce in the client some positive change, involving some corrective experience, across all therapeutic approaches. But he noted, too, that the nature of the interaction and the relative weight of each of these variables differ across theoretical orientations.

In general, behavioral and CBT approaches have understood and accepted the premise that an effective relationship provides the necessary context for any specific clinical intervention. Relational components, including warmth and empathy, may be necessary, but they are hardly sufficient. In CBT, therapists' provision of affirmation and PR does not manifest as the far-reaching, virtually unconditional type of acceptance that is emblematic of the PCA; in fact, clients engaged in CBT may feel that their therapist's penchant for challenging their thoughts and feelings is invalidating. Instead, the therapy relationship in behavioral and CBT approaches is often seen as serving to "encourage and reinforce clients for risk-taking like engaging in more effective between-session behavior" (Goldfried & Davila, 2005, p. 428).

Arguably, that contemporary cognitive or CBT therapist whose work is most consonant with Rogers's emphasis on PR in clinical work is Judith Beck. In her book outlining the basics of CBT, the second key principle noted is the requirement of a "sound therapeutic alliance," one established by demonstrating "warmth, empathy, caring, genuine regard, and competence" (J. S. Beck, 2011, p. 7). And J. S. Beck, like Goldfried before her, rejected the common myth that CBT, being a manualized treatment, is meant to be "cold and mechanical" (p. 19), dedicating a substantial portion of an early section of the book to providing what is essentially a manualized guide to Rogers's facilitative conditions, including that of PR:

> You will continuously demonstrate your commitment to and understanding of patients through your empathic statements, choice of words, tone of voice, facial expressions, and body language. As I tell my trainees, you strive to be a nice human being in the room with patients. You treat them the way you would like to be treated. You demonstrate empathy and accurate comprehension of their problems and ideas through your thoughtful questions, reflections, and statements, which leads to their feeling valued and understood. You will try to impart the following implicit (and sometimes explicit) messages, but only when you genuinely endorse them:
> "I care about you and value you."
> "I want to understand what you are experiencing and help you."
> "I'm confident we can work well together and that cognitive behavior therapy will help."
> "I'm not overwhelmed by your problems, even though you might be."
> "I've helped other patients much like you." (p. 18)

Beck noted, too, in a nod to Roger's call for congruence on the part of therapists, that the CBT practitioner must be genuine when expressing these feelings and thoughts to the patient and also noted that if this is challenging to the practitioner, additional support must be sought out to remedy this.

J. S. Beck (2011) further specified that CBT therapists must be alert to their patients' reactions and remain attuned to patients' experiences, which, in addition to helping the therapist structure future sessions, can also contribute to patients feeling more seen, honored, and valued. She also noted that although most patients respond positively to increased regard and warmth, not all do: "A patient may perceive you as being overly caring or too 'touchy-feely'" (p. 20). Part of Beck's conceptualization of PR is being respectful of specific patient sensitivities, adapting one's own style to be more compatible with what the patient perceives as genuinely supportive.

Judith Beck seems to have adopted some of her father's values and attitudes in regard to the importance of the therapeutic relationship, including the need for therapists to be supportive. The late Aaron T. Beck was the founder of cognitive therapy and someone recognized by the American Psychological Association as one of the five most influential psychotherapists of all time. In *Cognitive Therapy and the Emotional Disorders*, A. T. Beck (1979), like his daughter would later do, invoked Rogers in noting the importance of warmth, acceptance, and empathy in successful treatment outcomes.

Affirming these ideas and reminding readers that a study (Staples et al., 1975) showed that in comparison to psychoanalysts, behavior therapists actually conveyed more empathy and comparable warmth, Castonguay et al. (2018) argued that CBT "has a long history of endorsing warmth, empathy, and collaborative affiliation in theory, practice, and research" (p. 159). Their case example, that of a 25-year-old man with a skin-picking disorder, emphasized the role of the therapist's acceptance and validation in catalyzing the client's ability to alter his schema (i.e., that others were always judgmental, that he himself was not good enough) and engage far more effectively in the treatment.

Once again, though, it's important to note that whereas there are demonstrable elements of PR within the broad range of CBT treatments and significant emphasis on PR within some forms of CBT (e.g., cognitive therapy), these tend to be of secondary importance—essentially, context for more technical interventions. With some exceptions, these treatments do not regard PR or other Rogerian conditions as significant change agents in their own right, nor does their form of PR adopt a nonjudgmental, nondirective attitude as a feature of PR. From a humanistic—or, more specifically, person-centered—approach, there is a considerable distinction between the PR (affirmation) that may be conveyed in response to the behavior of a specifically desired action and the PR that is nonconditional and reflective of an overall attitude of acceptance of a person. Indeed, the PR afforded in consequence of a desired action is exactly what Rogers meant by "conditions of worth" and from his perspective and those of like-minded others, not the PR that individuals need in order to be truly self-accepting and thrive. Thus, while UPR is fairly anathema to CBT treatments, PR construed broadly is a powerful and relevant ingredient in the overall process of CBT, as clearly laid out by its most prominent advocates. The significant and demonstrable therapeutic benefits of CBT for many therapy patients with a wide range of presenting complaints is, for us, a potent argument in favor of taking a more expansive view of PR.

MARSHA LINEHAN AND VALIDATION

In her writings about DBT, Linehan's use of the term "validation" seems to come closer to Rogers's sense of PR than any other theorist's outside the person-centered orbit. According to Linehan (1993), the essence of validation is the therapist's communicating to the client that "her responses make sense and are understandable within her current life context or situation" (p. 222). Furthermore, wrote Linehan (1993), in validating the client, "the therapist actively accepts the client and communicates this acceptance to the client. The therapist takes the client's responses seriously and does not discount or trivialize them" (pp. 222–223). Consistent, too, with the views of Rogers, Linehan suggested that the therapist's validation facilitates changes that lead to therapeutic progress and the realization of a client's goals.

In fact, Linehan (1993) explicitly recognized how similar the concept of validation is to the concept of PR: "The person, rather than the constructs brought to the interaction by the therapist, is seen and countenanced. Validation used in this sense perhaps comes closest to the meaning of the term 'unconditional positive regard' used by Rogers (1959)" (p. 357). Like many theorists influenced by Rogers, she noted the potential for tension between the imperative for unconditional acceptance and the assumptions and practices of therapists of varying persuasions.

Further, like many of Rogers's followers, Linehan (1993) attempted to discriminate between validation and empathy. While noting the considerable overlap between these concepts, she also drew a distinction: "Although validation encompasses and requires empathy, it is more than empathy" (p. 355). For Rogers (1980), empathy is "perceiving the internal frame of reference of another [including its emotional components] with accuracy" (p. 141). In contrast, according to Linehan (1993), validation is the communication that the client's responses and patterns of behavior have inherent validity (p. 359). Thus, for Linehan, validation, especially in its more advanced forms (see the following), includes a component that Rogers doesn't consider necessary in the provision of PR: the therapist's explicit acknowledgment that what the client is saying is justified and rational within the client's worldview—that the client's words, feelings, and thoughts make sense.

Linehan posited six levels of validation within DBT. The first three levels reflect increasing degrees of empathy: from appearing interested (Stage 1) to accurately reflecting (Stage 2) to "mind reading" (Stage 3)—the latter in which therapists attempt to correctly articulate clients' unverbalized thoughts and feelings. In Stage 4, therapists communicate their understanding of clients' perceptions of the antecedents of their behavior; in addition, they validate clients' ideas about the necessity of their behaviors, even as they invalidate the wisdom or value of these behaviors. In Stage 5, therapists validate by attempting to find the "kernel of truth" in the client's experience. Finally, in Stage 6, at the level that Linehan termed "radical genuineness," validation occurs in the form of the therapist expressing belief in the client's capabilities in the present and the future. Whether deemed "validation" or "positive regard," at this stage, the therapist's genuine and direct words and actions reflect the sense that the client is a reasonable and effective individual.

In some ways, Linehan solved the problem of whether PR should include an explicitly validating component by suggesting that this attitude occurs on a continuum. However, to the extent that only the higher ends of her validation continuum contain elements of explicit confirmation and affirmation of the client's worthiness, Linehan implied that Rogers's emphasis on acceptance and nonjudgment may be insufficient for some clients' self-acceptance and healing. That said, we believe Linehan's greatest contribution to an expanded understanding of PR is her contention that acceptance and challenge can and should coexist—in other words, that clients need to be both validated and pushed. Linehan's position vis-à-vis clients, one that many therapists may feel comfortable adopting, is along the lines of "I accept and understand all that you do, and I absolutely challenge you to do better."

WILLIAM R. MILLER, UNCONDITIONAL LOVE (AGAPE), AND MOTIVATIONAL INTERVIEWING

One means of understanding the healing potential of PR is by invoking the concept of "agape" (unconditional love). William R. Miller (2000), a codeveloper (along with Stephen Rollnick) of motivational interviewing, has suggested that with rare exceptions (e.g., Erich Fromm), psychologists have overlooked the transformative powers of love in overcoming dysfunctional behavioral patterns. Miller wrote of struggling persistently with the question of what triggers change in clients, especially those with deep-rooted substance abuse issues who have long seemed refractory to attempts to alter their behavior. What seems to have finally made the difference? After analyzing multiple studies and ideas, Miller came to the realization that he had seen the phenomenon of sudden transformative experiences before—in "everyday life, where it is called *love*" (p. 11).

W. R. Miller (2000) suggested that the love he is referring to here is best embodied in the Greek word *agape*, a form of love often described as selfless, accepting, unlimited, and enduring. Of particular relevance to us is that Miller argued that the concept of agape is highly concordant with Rogers's facilitative conditions: "It is when a person experiences acceptance *as he or she really is* that change is facilitated" (p. 12). Miller expanded on his ideas by delineating five components of agape: *patience* (waiting, with no hurry, with the client), *selflessness* (a constant focus on the concerns of the client), *acceptance* (openness to whatever the client experiences), *hope* (belief in the client's potential), and *positive regard* itself (a respect for and valuing of the client as a person of worth). Although Miller named PR as one of the aspects of agape, all of these specified qualities can be seen as part of an omnibus view of PR.

"It is just possible," W. R. Miller (2000) wrote,

> that in ancient wisdom there lies a construct, lost for much of 20th century psychology, that will be of some value in organizing and interpreting emergent data on human change in the century ahead. Looking through this lens may point us in fruitful directions toward the understanding and refinement of healing love and not only in the context of psychotherapy. (p. 15)

In invoking the concept of agape, Miller seems to be suggesting that contemporary clinicians should be more accepting of that aspect of PR that Rogers referred to as "nonpossessive love."

CONCLUSION

What we hope has emerged from these synopses is an appreciation of the wide range of therapies in which some aspect of PR is integral to the values and processes of that system. What we hope has also become apparent is that whereas some aspects of Rogers's ways of defining this attitude remain—support, caring, acceptance, and warmth all come to mind—this concept, like most concepts in the social sciences, has been subject to revision by subsequent generations of therapists. The specific nature of PR—the ways in which therapists manifest this attitude emotionally and behaviorally—seems now to have expanded, and, we argue, this is a positive development that has allowed more therapy practitioners and clients to access and benefit from the powerful and ground-breaking ideas of Rogers. "I am large," Walt Whitman (1855) wrote, "I contain multitudes" ("Song of Myself," Section 51).

Some of the material in this chapter points toward the need for therapists to be particularly mindful of conveying PR at certain times during treatment (e.g., when alliance ruptures are emerging). But most of the theoretical and clinical adaptations noted here are in the direction of the therapist's more active and explicit conveyance of PR. Yalom advocates for consistent therapist self-disclosure and overt affirmation of regard for clients; Winnicott insists on the need for a therapist to be empathic, caring, and responsive; Bowlby and Kohut suggest that interpretations of client behavioral patterns can be seen as sensitively responsive, affirming actions; Wachtel and other relationally oriented psychodynamic therapists maintain that within the overall matrix of a therapist's support and affirmation, there should be ample space for a therapist's questions, challenges, and interpretations; Judith and Aaron Beck promote overt expressions of support and caring while de-emphasizing the need for a therapist's unconditional acceptance; Linehan suggests that acceptance and nonjudgment may be insufficient for some clients (e.g., those diagnosed with borderline personality disorder) and, moreover, that acceptance and challenge should not be seen as incompatible therapist actions but rather in dialectical terms; and Miller implies that therapists should not shy away from appropriating the healing power of nonpossessive love. We concur with virtually all of these ideas and believe that therapists of all theoretical persuasions should consider incorporating at least some of these practices within their own clinical model of treatment.

In the next chapter, we examine the ways in which PR is manifest in several nontherapeutic contexts. We discuss a contemporary of Carl Rogers—Fred Rogers—who seems to have embodied so much of what Carl Rogers meant by "positive regard." We look, too, at how PR seems to be played out in our current era, focusing our attention on individuals nominated as being highly positively regarding by graduate students in psychology and on the ways in which PR is conveyed through social media. In looking into the nature of PR in circumstances outside of the treatment room, we can learn more about the universality of PR as well as the diverse ways in which our clients might be capable of receiving PR within the therapeutic relationship.

5 POSITIVE REGARD OUTSIDE PSYCHOTHERAPY

Another Rogers, Personal Relationships, and Social Media

The world needs a sense of worth, and it will achieve it only by its people feeling that they are worthwhile.

—Fred Rogers

While the work of Carl Rogers was geared primarily toward studying processes within the therapy relationship, the theory he developed was far broader in scope. In fact, Rogers (1959) viewed the therapeutic relationship as "just one instance of interpersonal relationship" (p. 236) and laid out his facilitative conditions as universal. Whether in a home, educational, or social setting, these circumstances, if met, could promote constructive personality change within the context of a variety of nurturing relationships. Many of us have been fortunate enough to experience the transformative power of positive regard (PR) in our extratherapy relationships. A teacher's gentle attention and affirmation can make us feel truly seen and inspire us to attain goals we hadn't thought possible, and the unwavering love and support of a parent, sibling, best friend, or romantic partner can promote incredible resilience and deep healing through life's challenges.

https://doi.org/10.1037/0000312-006
Understanding and Enhancing Positive Regard in Psychotherapy: Carl Rogers and Beyond, by B. A. Farber, J. Y. Suzuki, and D. Ort

PR can be applied in broader contexts as well—for example, in our public discourse and on social media. In this chapter, we observe PR at work as a potent healing force in the world outside of the treatment room. First, we review the work of public-television luminary Fred Rogers, who, in addition to sharing a name with the founder of person-centered therapy, grounded his career in an ethos that was uncannily similar to Carl Rogers's notion of PR. Next, we amplify the voices of clinical psychology graduate students as they reflect on the most and least positively regarding individuals in their personal lives. The insights these psychologically minded individuals offer into their personal relationships dovetail with the clinical and theoretical ideas we have reviewed about PR, while adding additional dimension and perspective. Finally, we examine applications of PR in the internet era, considering how now-ubiquitous forms of digital communication have shaped, reinforced, and altered the expression of and the need for PR.

Examining the ways in which PR is conveyed outside of psychotherapy may suggest new ways of conveying this attitude within a treatment setting. It may also further our understanding of which specific aspects of PR most resonate with a wide sample of individuals, some of whom will surely at some point be psychotherapy clients.

FRED (MISTER) ROGERS: "IT'S A BEAUTIFUL DAY IN THE NEIGHBORHOOD"

Fred Rogers (1928–2003) began working in children's television in 1951; *Mister Rogers' Neighborhood* ran on television from 1968 to 2001. He hosted, starred in, and wrote most of the material for the 895 episodes of that program, including the many songs. Each show had a theme, many focused on fraught contemporary or familial issues that children might be experiencing: illness, death, sibling rivalry, divorce, new family members, and beginning or changing schools. Mister Rogers believed that the principles that guided his message to children applied equally to adults and to society at large. As we note shortly, he also dealt, in his own way, with civil rights issues; notably, too, he devoted one show in 1968 to coping with the assassination of Robert Kennedy.

The shared name is just a coincidence—they are not related—but it is curious that the contemporary figure outside of the realm of psychology whose work reflected most closely the Rogerian ethos of PR was Fred Rogers. They were both warm, gentle figures with difficult, somewhat lonely childhoods—both with a background in the ministry; both interested in child development; both focused on the importance of acceptance of others and of loving relationships;

and both offering humane, empathic, nonconformist visions of how to help others grow and become their best, true selves. Before turning to psychology, Dr. Rogers studied for the ministry; Mister Rogers was ordained as a Presbyterian minister. Carl's client-centered approach stood in great contrast to the formal and hierarchical structure of the then-dominant psychoanalytic community; Fred's leisurely, slow-paced style of modeling social-emotional lessons to children offered a strong counterpoint to the fast-paced and cognitively focused world of *Sesame Street* and the frenetic, often-violent world of children's cartoons. One of their biographers noted that her subject emphasized the values of "patience, reflection, and silence in a noisy world" (King, 2018, p. 9); that happened to be said of Fred, but one can easily imagine it being applied to Carl as well.

Both Carl and Fred showed great respect for the inherent wisdom of their clientele, and both were parodied for their supposed naivete and inability to accept or confront the more sordid aspects of life. Both believed in the critical importance of understanding and expressing one's feelings. Carl's emphasis was on actively listening for and accepting the feelings and emotions behind clients' words. He believed that such actions on the part of the therapist would lead to clients' ability to recognize, express, and accept their own feelings. At Fred's 1969 testimony before a Senate subcommittee that was considering cutting funding for public television, he, too, emphasized the connection between the ability of individuals to express and accept their feelings and the emergence of self-worth:

> This is what I give. I give an expression of care every day to each child, to help him realize that he is unique. . . . I feel that if we in public television can only make it clear that feelings are mentionable and manageable, we will have done a great service for mental health. (The Fred Rogers Company, 2018)

Both believed greatly in the importance of nonjudgmental acceptance, of nonpossessive love, of no imposed "conditions of worth" from caregivers. Fred Rogers (2019) attributed this sentiment to his grandfather, remembering his grandfather saying to him, "Freddy, I like you, just the way you are" (p. 1). On his show, he would often sing a song that expresses nearly perfectly the essence of what Carl Rogers meant by "positive regard": "It's you I like, it's not the things you wear/It's not the way you do your hair—but it's you I like." And Fred, much like Carl, believed greatly in the potential of positive regard (though without using that phrase) to make a difference in the lives of those to whom it was conveyed. His description of supportive, caring, and highly responsive listening—here articulated when he was the commencement speaker at Dartmouth College in 2002—differs from his psychotherapist namesake, but the essence of their message is much the same: "From the time you were very little, you've had people who have smiled you into smiling, people who have talked you into talking, sung you into singing, loved you into loving" (The Fred Rogers Company, 2018). Fred Rogers was said to exude "radical kindness" (Heller, cited by Junod, 2019), an attribute that could easily have been applied to Carl Rogers as well.

Palmer and Carr (1991) wrote a short article 3 decades ago comparing Carl Rogers and Fred Rogers and concluding, as we have, that the concordance between them was remarkable: "Their sensitivities, their values, and their talents produced career trajectories firmly committed to children, to self-acceptance, and the positive gifts and potential in our lives and in the lives of those around us" (p. 43). Furthermore, these authors noted, both of these extraordinary public figures were committed to the overarching idea that we all need to be accepted for who we are.

Both also took strong stands against racial inequality, guided by the belief that the need for empathy and acceptance extends beyond the bounds of family relationships to society and humanity as a whole. Carl devoted much of the later years of his professional career to attempting to heal racial and ethnic wounds in Northern Ireland and South Africa, efforts that led to his being nominated for the Nobel Peace Prize. At a time (1969) when racial tensions were heightened and swimming pools in the United States were still segregated, Fred Rogers famously invited Officer Clemmons, a Black police officer on the show, to join him in dunking their feet into a small, plastic wading pool. Years later, in 2018, Clemmons told a Vermont news website, "It was a definite call to social action on Fred's part. That was his way of speaking about race relations in America" (Kettler, 2020). More generally, though, both Fred and Carl Rogers were modest individuals, and each believed their essential message of believing in the goodness of others just might lead to a better world.

To provide further evidence of the great similarities in their thinking, especially in regard to their ideas about empathy and PR, Exhibit 5.1 lists some of the sayings of Fred Rogers and Carl Rogers. But we've purposely omitted from this exhibit which of these two figures articulated which of these thoughts. That information, some of which we suspect will seem surprising, is provided at the end of this chapter.

The work of Mister Rogers offers a valuable sense of the expansiveness of PR—how instrumental it is in not only our family relationships but also our connections with our friends, neighbors, and communities—and especially across lines of diversity and difference. In a similar fashion, therapists can consider the ripple effects of PR within their clients' lives and beyond: not just the possibility that a client lacked sufficient PR from early caregivers but also inquiring about places and relationships in which PR was more available

EXHIBIT 5.1. Thoughts About Empathy and Positive Regard From Carl Rogers and Fred Rogers

- "Nothing can replace the influence of unconditional love in the life of a child."
- "Listening is where love begins."
- "There are times when explanations, no matter how reasonable, just don't seem to help."
- "Most of us strive mightily to be perfectly lovable in the eyes of those we love. What those eyes tell us while we are infants are the important messages we get about the value of being who we are."
- "When we love a person, we accept him or her exactly as is: the lovely with the unlovely, the strong with the fearful, the true mixed in with the façade, and of course, the only way we can do is by accepting ourselves that way."
- "Listening and trying to understand the needs of those we would communicate with seems to me the essential prerequisite of any communication. And we might as well aim for *real* communication."
- "Honesty linked with love is the most important response in any relationship."
- "A person can grow to his or her fullest capacity only in mutually caring relationships with others."
- "Showing an active interest in what a child is doing is sometimes the best compliment of all."
- "We all need to feel that we have gifts to give that are acceptable and valued."
- "One mother with a child who had been terribly frightened all the time told us, 'I've come to understand that, like everyone else, Nathan needs acceptance, understanding, tolerance, patience, and love—and then he does have the resources for dealing with life.'"
- "Almost always, when a person realizes he has been deeply heard, his eyes moisten. I think in some real sense he is weeping for joy. It is as though he were saying, 'Thank God, somebody heard me.'"

Note. Quote attributions can be found at the end of the chapter.

or may have had a powerful compensatory effect, whether in childhood or in the present day. In this sense, therapists may benefit from conceptualizing the PR they offer their clients as potentially having broad reverberations—that clients, having been positively regarded, become positively regarding to those they now encounter.

We believe that the extraordinary popularity of Fred Rogers provides further, "on the ground" evidence of the salience of PR for nearly all individuals. Like Carl Rogers, he consistently expressed great interest in others and greatly valued and accepted their feelings. What else might a therapist interested in enhancing PR with clients extrapolate from the career of Fred Rogers? Perhaps to actively look for the good in others; to value silence and soft speech; to provide self-care as a way of modeling the need for self-worth and as a means of expressing one's investment in the work and one's care for clients; and, especially important in these times, to appreciate differences—different identities, lifestyles, family arrangements, religions, and cultures.

ATTRIBUTES OF THE MOST POSITIVELY REGARDING PEOPLE KNOWN TO GRADUATE STUDENTS IN PSYCHOLOGY

In the early stages of developing our research protocols, our team often draws on the wisdom and insights of a readily available sample—clinical psychology graduate students—and occasionally the results of these pilot studies are interesting and rich enough to report on their own merits. To begin to better understand PR outside of the client–therapist relationship, we asked a group of master's and doctoral students within our university to describe an individual they believed was "best at providing positive regard" and to elaborate on the specific characteristics and behaviors of this person. Conversely, we asked them to describe someone who was "least good at providing positive regard." We believed we could learn more about PR by identifying characteristics of not only positive models of this attribute but negative models, as well.

Although generalizing the results of these data—drawn from students familiar with the work of Rogers and the concept of the therapeutic alliance—is unwarranted, the results of this informal study indicated a significant overlap in the way PR was perceived and experienced in both clinical and nonclinical settings. There may well be a consistency to what individuals truly want and value from important others in their lives.

Some of the frequently noted characteristics, with examples, of individuals considered by graduate students in psychology to be especially good at providing PR follow:

Honesty

"What is most important to me, and what I appreciate most about my friend, is that when she does not know something, she admits it. She rarely puts up a front, and in this way, I feel a strong sense of realness and genuineness in her."

Acceptance/A Nonjudgmental Attitude

"When I shared my distress over my car accident with friends and family members they told me I was overreacting—the car would get fixed and I should focus on how lucky I was that I was not injured. However, when I shared this experience with my significant other, he didn't mention anything like that to me. He made me feel like it was okay to be upset and he allowed me the space to express whatever emotions I needed to express without feeling foolish."

"My father is the kind of person that everyone wants to share their story with because he hardly judges people and instead is always kind and willing to listen."

Empathy

"When I'm embarrassed or ashamed of something I've done or experienced, it always feels safe to give T a call. It feels safe, because as a close friend he can really climb into my shoes and see things through my eyes without judgment."

"When I was struggling with my marriage, and experienced a draining amount of self-doubt and worry, my best friend did not victimize or catastrophize—instead, she provided a safe space for me in which she tried to better understand and acknowledge my feelings. Her ability to do this helped me remain calm during this crisis."

Affirmation

"During our conversations, when I'm doubtful of whether I will be a good enough therapist or not, MT reminds me of my existing qualities—'you're so warm, comforting and accepting, obviously you'll be a great psychologist one day.'"

Ability to Reframe Weaknesses as Strengths

"What I so appreciate about my partner is the way he helps me reframe aspects of myself that I see as negative to positive. For example, when I was feeling down on myself for being overly sensitive, he said, 'I think the fact that you're sensitive makes you a very compassionate person.'"

Ability to Listen

"She is a very engaged and focused listener. No matter how long our conversation, she maintains eye contact and pays attention to what I am saying. She always sits facing towards me. The most important thing is that she never interrupts me or judges what I am saying. Instead, she asks open-ended questions to try to better understand various aspects of what I am saying."

"The most prominent way she makes me feel positively regarded is the way she quietly listens to me talk—and sometimes I can go on for quite a while—and she never interrupts. While she listens, it feels as if she is really internalizing what I am saying, which feels really important to me."

Consistency

"My friend A is an example of someone who is very good at providing positive regard. What makes her so good at this, is that unlike many of my friends, she is consistent in her provision of positive regard."

Recollection of Significant Personal Details

"She remembers the names of all the people I interact with, my school mates, my professors, and my colleagues at work."

Interest in the Whole Person

"My friend always demonstrates a genuine interest in me 'as a whole person'—she's not just interested in one aspect of my life."

Again, most of these qualities are quite consistent with the writings of Rogers and his colleagues about the nature and provision of PR. PR, according to our small sample of millennial-age graduate student respondents, is not defined by offering compliments or simply being nice; it is far more about an overarching sense of acceptance, interest, encouragement, and emotional holding. Interestingly, too, none of our respondents included "challenging" in their descriptions of positively regarding individuals. Whereas some theorists (see Chapter 4) have suggested that challenging or confronting a client could be considered a valid aspect of PR, none of our current sample expressed that thought. In a similar fashion, Ben-Eliyahu et al. (2021) found that 15-year-olds believed that positively regarding mentors were honest, dependable, and good listeners; these positively regarding adults were also seen as remembering statements from previous conversations and appreciating (laughing at) teens' jokes. However, in contrast to our graduate student sample, these teens suggested that positively regarding adults could be somewhat challenging, at least in terms of holding them to higher standards vis-à-vis their peers.

ATTRIBUTES OF THE LEAST POSITIVELY REGARDING PEOPLE KNOWN TO GRADUATE STUDENTS IN PSYCHOLOGY

Although we imagined that our exercise asking these graduate students to describe a person or persons who were "least good" at providing PR would yield accounts of hostile, antisocial, overly critical, or narcissistic individuals, most of our respondents described reasonably well-meaning individuals who seemingly provided some form of caring but in a form that was compromised or significantly flawed in some way.

Conditionality

Many of our respondents alluded to the hurtful features of PR that feels conditional. In some way or another, they echoed Rogerian ideas about the wounding aspects of conditions of worth—of being affirmed but only when their behavior was consonant with another's needs or values. The message inherent in many of these narratives was "I would rather not be supported or accepted or affirmed at all than feel manipulated." This sentiment evokes not only Rogers and Winnicott ("false self") but brings to mind an incident in one of the filmed interviews in Shostrom's (1965) *Three Approaches to Psychotherapy*. Gloria, the client in each of these demonstration interviews, met for 30-minute sessions with Rogers, Albert Ellis, and Fritz Perls. Her work with Perls was especially provocative. Following a barrage of disparaging remarks from Perls, Gloria exclaimed,

> I feel like you're telling me the only way you'd respect me as a human being is if I'm aggressive and forceful and strong . . . I'd be scared to death to cry in front of you. I feel like you'd laugh at me and call me a phony. I feel you don't accept my weak side. (Shostrom, 1965)

This general phenomenon also calls to mind the work of Alice Miller (1981/1997), whose book *The Drama of the Gifted Child: The Search for the True Self* (originally published as *Prisoners of Childhood: The Drama of the Gifted Child and the Search for the True Self*) postulated that children who are especially attuned to and susceptible to acting in accord with parental needs ultimately experience a terrible emptiness, a loss of a deep sense of self. It also calls to mind the wise lyrics of Paul Simon (1983) in the song "Hearts and Bones": "And tell me why, why won't you love me, for who I am, where I am?"

Many therapists also believe that adults who grew up under conditions of worth continue to be vigilant and even suspicious of praise that feels contaminated by ulterior motives. Some narratives among our sample that express this perspective follow:

> "My parents only provide positive regard when I am doing what they think I should be doing. This feels very conditional. I know it doesn't come from a lack of love. . . . But in the end, I am left without enough positive regard, and I often feel I need to change my plans to align with theirs in order to receive more positive regard."

> "In order for us to be friends I had to always meet certain standards and expectations . . . hers was a caring that lasted as long as it satisfied her own needs."

Acting Judgmentally

There were several other astute observations from these respondents regarding the ways in which apparent instances of PR became corrupted. The narratives here speak to how PR cannot be truly conveyed by a person who is a poor listener and/or judgmental:

> "Even though my aunt might appear to be positively regarding by maintaining eye contact and active listening, she interrupts me a lot and appears to jump to judgmental conclusions. She tries to show how well she knows me by finishing my sentences and giving me advice before I even finish sharing."

> "Instead of listening hard to me or offering support or a new way of understanding myself, she [my friend] listens quickly and then tries to fix the problem for me. When she does this [gives advice too quickly] it makes me feel like she's dismissive of my feelings."

Pairing Affirmation With Criticism

"Yes, but" is a phenomenon that frustrates many individuals when arguing, or even speaking cordially, with another. This kind of communication too often feels like a tease, with the "yes" part containing an affirmation or message of support but also an implicit justification for the criticism or judgment that inevitably follows. Thus, another frequently noted attribute of those who are poor at providing PR is their penchant for pairing affirmation with criticism.

> "While my relative is very good at remembering details of my life, she often uses my past to point out previous mistakes that I made. For example, when I was struggling in my romantic relationship, she said, 'I know you have a very kind and generous heart, but don't make the same mistake you made with your previous boyfriend, don't give too much of yourself to someone who will walk away.' In these cases, her compliments and ability to remember my experiences make me feel as if her praise is just a way for her to balance her criticism."

Invalidating

A somewhat less toxic, but still quite distressing, variation on this theme involves the person who eschews overt criticism but nonetheless cannot hear the pain or distress of the other. This insensitivity or nonacceptance of certain aspects of another often occurs with parents in a manner reminiscent of Linehan's (1993) notion of "invalidation." Our respondents evoked images of a mom or dad who, while stating unconditional love for them, nevertheless could not or would not allow them to express any sad or self-deprecating feelings. "You shouldn't feel that way" is the essence of this kind of failure to provide PR.

> "I recall that it was very difficult for me to share my feelings or opinions with her. The few times that I tried, she would brush my worries aside by telling me that there are bigger things that one should worry about. In order to gain her appreciation, I would always feel the need to say certain things in front of her, be a certain way."

> "My mother is a typical 'tiger mom.' She loves me—that is very clear—but she is always focused on helping me improve. . . . For example, if I communicate that something is wrong, she responds by saying something like, 'You will be fine, your problems are nothing compared to what I dealt with at your age.'"

This situation can also happen with friends:

> "She [my friend] is the type of person who can physically be there, but whenever I turn to her for support, she instead provides me with a laundry list of positives in my life that I should be thankful for. This leads me to feel like my complaints and stressors are insignificant, and I feel like a fool for needing support."

Inconsistency and Insincerity

Several respondents also remarked how unsatisfied they felt when PR was inconsistently offered by someone close to them:

> "He was inconsistently positively regarding, which made it feel very superficial. Sometimes he would be overly engaged and seem very interested in me and what I had to say, other times he didn't seem to care at all. These contradictions led me to feel confused about whether he really cared."

Some respondents also noted that they couldn't trust or believe others' efforts at conveying PR because those efforts felt insincere—or what Rogers would have deemed nongenuine. In a similar vein, Daniel Stern (1985), in his work on mothers' attunement to children, noted that responsiveness to a child's message was sometimes performed in a perfunctory, inauthentic manner. Stern remarked that "as every parent knows, your heart can't always be in it" (p. 217). But there is, of course, a difference between the inevitability of occasionally not being fully present to the needs of another—a phenomenon that is usually understood and accepted—and consistent half-hearted or insincere efforts to acknowledge, support, and care for another. The latter is the cause of many relational dissolutions, as well as the basis for much humor. An oft-shared contemporary meme: "Are you really listening or just waiting for your turn to speak?" Or, similarly, a classic dad joke: "My wife just stopped and said, 'You weren't even listening, were you?' I thought, *Hmm, that's a pretty strange way to start a conversation*." Two examples of this phenomenon from our sample of students follow:

> "He [my roommate] was sociable, friendly, and at first seemed like he cared about the events that were transpiring in my life. However, there was something inauthentic about the way he attempted to provide me with positive regard. For example, he repeatedly asked me the same sort of general questions, which made me feel like he wasn't truly listening to me."

> "Before even having a good understanding of my situation, she would say things like, 'I really feel you,' or, 'I completely understand.' She did this constantly, jumping to provide PR before really listening or understanding what I was experiencing. This made me feel like her PR was insincere, and eventually I stopped sharing my experiences with her."

PR, understood broadly by our respondents and well beyond the parameters of Rogers's formulations, can be rendered in a fashion that feels somehow impersonal or inauthentic, making it feel less about the person to whom it is directed and more about the person articulating these sentiments. In this regard, several respondents noted that the seeming PR of their significant others—most often in the form of overt compliments—felt like it was signifying either the virtue of their partner or an impending request. Similarly, some respondents indicated that the PR conveyed by their parents often felt like parental bragging or was implicitly affirming of their parents' virtues rather than their own.

> "When my father does provide positive regard to me, it typically is in front of other people. He'll say something like, 'You are a great friend, daughter, student' but I really don't appreciate that he does this in front of others. Not only do I not like this because I am a private person and I feel uncomfortable in the moment, but it also makes me feel like he has ulterior motives—either he is doing it in front of others to make it look like he is always so complimentary, or he is bragging about me."

What also stood out for us, in going through these narratives, was the extent to which most respondents rationalized why so-and-so was poor at providing PR: "My parents never learned it from their own parents," "My culture doesn't emphasize these values," "My parents (or friends or significant other) really meant well by providing advice," "Everybody is in so much of a hurry now; maybe that's all anyone really should expect." The overall message here, that we all need to become accustomed to imperfect efforts—even excuse them—perhaps speaks to why therapists' consistent and sometimes-successful efforts to provide PR may feel so potent and healing.

POSITIVE REGARD ON SOCIAL MEDIA

Although the internet was in its infancy when Rogers died, and he could not have imagined the extent to which computer-mediated communication (CMC) would come to dominate our daily lives, we suspect he would not have been surprised by the extent to which PR remains an essential need served by our interactions online. PR is inherently relational, requiring communication of some mix of respect, acceptance, care, interest, warmth, and support by one party to another. Virtually all online domains—including email, texting, social media, videoconferencing, and gaming—offer means by which users can convey their own brand of PR to friends, acquaintances, or even strangers. These means are not exactly of the sort that Rogers had in mind when he wrote of the ways in which therapists could and should be positively regarding to their clients. Clearly, the nature and aims of the personal interaction in the therapeutic dyad and in connections forged or maintained via social media are dramatically different. Still, even with the constraints of social media, there are some novel and meaningful ways that users have found to provide forms of PR—or at least approximations thereof—that Rogers might well be impressed with. For our purposes, though, understanding how PR is provided on social media is important because it likely influences the ways that some psychotherapy clients, especially digital natives, will respond to the specific nature of the PR provided by their therapist. Moreover, with the increased clinical use of digital platforms and CMC, it is especially important for therapists to understand the distinct ways that PR may be communicated across these channels.

Some context first: Social media should not be regarded as a monolith. Platforms such as Facebook, Twitter, LinkedIn, YouTube, and Instagram (to name only a handful) operate under different customs, rules, and technical functionalities. Communicating PR on these platforms is similar to communicating respect and care in different countries: The specific actions and language may be different, but the gist is similar. There is, however, one significant common factor across social media that is important to note. The expression of every emotion or attitude on social media, including the expression of PR, is affected by what is known as the *online disinhibition effect* (Suler, 2004)—the tendency of individuals to act in a disinhibited (i.e., less restrained) manner, either in a "toxic" or "benign" direction. The directionality and nature of online disinhibition can be influenced by situational factors, including how anonymous and invisible a user feels and how "real" the users on the other side of the interaction feel (Suler, 2004). But sometimes these factors operate in nonintuitive ways. For example, Hollenbaugh and Everett (2013) found that visual identifiers of blog authors led to more disclosure of personal information in writing—somewhat contrary to intuition that people would be more reserved when they are able to be visually identified.

These situational factors are relevant because every social media platform offers its own signature blend of cues and interpersonal features that create unique social experiences. For example, on Facebook, individual users are (usually) highly identifiable: Every comment or post has the author's name and profile picture attached, as if wearing a digital identification card at all times. On Instagram, however, it is not uncommon for users to go by pseudonyms, though visual identifiers are still common. On Snapchat, users commonly go by pseudonyms, and visual identifiers contained in messages disappear, after seconds, without a trace. And on 4chan, commonly regarded as one of the rougher and more aggressive platforms on the internet, users are truly anonymous, with not even distinct usernames to differentiate one poster from the next. Thus, users may feel more inhibited on Facebook, where everyone "knows" who they are, versus on 4chan, where anything they say (including an expletive-laced insult) cannot be traced to their nononline selves.

With the backdrop of users acting under the sometimes slight, sometimes powerful effects of online disinhibition, we now turn to the four ways we believe that PR is typically expressed over social media: approval, endorsement, expressive support, and explicit connection.

Approval is a simple action that is achievable with a click of a button on most major social media platforms—specifically, the like button. Like buttons are present on Facebook (the like/love button), Instagram (the heart button), YouTube (the like video and like comment buttons), Reddit (the upvote button), and LinkedIn (the like button). When a user clicks these buttons, they are communicating to the original poster something akin to "I have heard what you have expressed, and I approve of what you wrote." The specific meaning may be slightly different based on the context. It could mean something more like "I sympathize with what you, the poster, have communicated," "I congratulate you on what you have communicated," or "I find what you wrote entertaining or insightful." As Pounds et al. (2018) observed,

> Facebook's salient "liking" option is used frequently in the group and may provide a nonverbal marker of positive regard, though the multiple functions of the Like response means it cannot be said to always unequivocally convey agreement or endorsement. Nevertheless, for some contributors receiving Likes may be experienced as adding a generally "approving" and, therefore, supportive dimension to the interactional environment. (p. 42)

The specific meaning of the approval can be more clearly communicated on some platforms, such as Facebook or LinkedIn, where users can specify that they are laughing, celebrating, deeming a comment insightful, offering heartfelt sympathy, or having another emotional reaction. For the most part, these users are expressing support and acceptance of another, hallmarks of how Rogers framed the communication of PR. However, to the extent that this form of approval contains an element of explicit endorsement or evaluation (e.g., suggesting that a user's political comment is wise), it seeps into the controversy that surrounds the legitimacy of explicit affirmation as an aspect of PR.

Perhaps the largest variety of approval actions is found on Reddit, a social media site where users operate anonymously under pseudonyms. In addition to the upvote button, users can also show larger levels of approval of posts or comments on posts by conferring special awards, most famously "Reddit Gold," which costs the awarder a small amount of money that goes to the website and highlights the awarded post or comment to other users. While these approval actions can convey PR, a similar type of button can be used to instead convey a lack of PR (or disapproval) on certain platforms (e.g., the angry or laughing reactions on Facebook, the dislike button on YouTube, the downvote button on Reddit). In addition to indicating PR, approval buttons are such easy and versatile ways to engage with others that they often play a critical role in helping these platforms determine what content is most appealing to users, so that they can show it more quickly to other users.

Endorsement is another expression of PR, one that can be seen as the next level of approval: It is approving of what a poster says to such a high degree that it is taken on by the user and passed along to their own network. It is the equivalent of saying to another person, "What you have said deserves to be heard by others, and I will help make that happen." This is achievable on several platforms with the click of a button: the share button on Facebook, the retweet button on Twitter, the add post to your story button on Instagram, and the pin comment button on YouTube. Again, the specific meanings may be different based on the context, and this action of endorsement can often be accompanied by approval or with expressive support, such as commentary on why the endorsement is being given—for example, "Everyone should read about Ken's brave experience" or "I just wanted to share this smart perspective my niece wrote about climate change." Endorsement often carries more weight or greater PR than approval, as the user who endorses is choosing to share their expression of PR with their own community. It is worth noting that, similar to online indications of approval, actions signifying "unendorsement" or ridicule can be performed via the same mechanisms as actions of endorsement, though this almost always requires clarification in commentary. For example, a person can share an acquaintance's Facebook post but with the caption "Look at how dumb my coworker is."

Expressive support cannot be done with a simple click of a button, which perhaps makes it more meaningful to the recipient than actions that can be done quickly and easily. Expressive support is commonly communicated either as stand-alone posts to another user's profile (e.g., on Facebook or YouTube) or as replies to a post or comment that another user made (e.g., on Facebook, YouTube, Instagram, Twitter, LinkedIn, Reddit). Expressive support is, by definition, unique to the expresser, unlike actions that can be done with the push of a button. This form of PR also stands out more to onlooking users than do button pushes. Expressive support indicates that the expresser is not only supportive but willing to go an extra step to show it. On a social media post such as a wedding photo that has received dozens or hundreds of approvals or likes, expressive support could take the form of a comment like "So happy for you both! Much love!" For a post commemorating the passing of a loved one, expressive support could include an empathic statement, such as "So sorry for your loss," or a related anecdote about the deceased. Expressive support could also take the form of coming to a friend's or unknown person's aid in an online confrontation. In an aggressive Facebook political debate, a person using expressive support to help an embattled friend might comment, "I feel like a lot of the people commenting on this post might be intentionally misunderstanding what you are saying. But I think your original post was very well said!" In a high school public cyberbullying episode, an acquaintance might be supportive and caring by defending the target of the bullying or by attacking the bullies. Again, whereas expressive support on social media may include some form of explicit judgment or evaluation (e.g., "well played," "great job," "you look terrific") that Rogers eschewed, we've noted that many theorists both inside and outside the person-centered tradition have argued for the legitimacy of these types of expressions within the overall concept of PR.

Explicit connection is usually accomplished with the click of a button and is an "ask" for placement in a user's social media network. Different platforms achieve explicit connection through button-press actions with platform-specific names—for example, "add friend" (Facebook), "follow" (Twitter, Facebook, and Instagram), "add" (Snapchat), "connect" (LinkedIn), and "subscribe" (YouTube). Explicit connection requires one party to initiate a request to connect to another and, generally, for the other party to explicitly accept that request. Some platforms do not require explicit acceptance of the request, as connection is confirmed automatically (e.g., Twitter, YouTube, Instagram, if the account is open to the public). The establishment of explicit connection can communicate a desire for an established, ongoing relationship between two parties—though explicit online connections may often simply correspond to already established offline connections. But a request for an explicit connection can also communicate a less intense request, such as "I would like to see more of your posts on this platform" or "I would like to grow my network, so I will reach out to you with the expectation that you will reciprocate, though there is no obligation." The person receiving the explicit connection may feel valued and acknowledged. Some platforms and/or users do require explicit acceptance of the request for explicit connection, which makes reciprocity a likely part of the expression of PR.

The opposite of explicit connection is explicit disconnection, but this can often be done by degrees. Not accepting a request for connection may be seen as explicit disconnection (e.g., not accepting a friend request on Facebook or a follow request on Instagram) and communicates something like "I am not interested in a relationship with you, even though you would like that." Removing an established connection through unfollowing, unfriending, unsubscribing, or blocking is also a form of explicit disconnection, though it may not always be clear to the recipient that they have lost the connection. Such an action of explicit disconnection would communicate something like "I am no longer interested in having a relationship with you" or "I am no longer interested in what you have to say in the future." *Ghosting*, which is when a person suddenly stops responding to communications from a particular person, often involves explicit disconnection on several platforms.

PERSONAL RELATIONSHIPS, SOCIAL MEDIA, AND POSITIVE REGARD

Members of romantic and platonic dyads today—especially those in the Gen X, millennial, and Gen Z age groups—tend to make frequent use of CMC. "Computer-mediated communication" is a broad term that includes all forms of electronic instant messaging—a feature of most social media platforms—including texts, private messages, and emails. CMC differs in significant ways from face-to-face (FtF) communication in that the latter provides ample opportunities for verbal and prosodic cues (the rhythm, tone, and sound of speech), nonverbal cues (e.g., body language, including facial expressions), and proxemic cues (how physically close two people are from each other). Nevertheless, there are still multiple means by which PR can be expressed to a specific other through CMC (O'Sullivan et al., 2004).

Personalness focuses on making the recipient of CMC feel seen as an individual. Personalized attentiveness from the "source" to the "receiver" is key and can be displayed by remembering and using names, integrating knowledge of the person while communicating, and using those channels (media) that the recipient prefers. The first and second elements here are common to FtF conveyance of PR (including in the psychotherapeutic context), but the third, switching to "richer channels," is unique to CMC.

Marshall McLuhan's oft-quoted phrase "the medium is the message" (McLuhan & Fiore, 1967) is relevant here, as the choice and timing of a communication channel can provide positive (or negative) relational cues to the recipient, such as by using a medium that the recipient has a stated preference for (e.g., "Please call me, I much prefer to talk over the phone than text").

Engagement is about "indicating attentiveness and practicing responsiveness to receivers" (O'Sullivan et al., 2004). Although this tack is consistent with conveying PR in FtF situations, the mechanisms by which attentiveness and responsiveness are shown in CMC are different. The ambiguity surrounding when messages are read and responded to creates more uncertainty around the timing ("chronemics") of CMC interactions. Studies exploring chronemic norms in asynchronous CMC have highlighted the ways in which the speed of response to a message informs the recipient's perception of the responder's level of regard for them (Kalman & Rafaeli, 2011; Walther & Tidwell, 1995).

Responding quickly to messages makes recipients feel like they are important and worth the time of the sender, a subtle signaling of PR (Fehr, 2003). And, since other activities will most likely get in the way of prompt responding, another PR-like element here is the acknowledgment of interruptions, such as "I have to run to class now, but I'll text you later!" or "Hey, I'm going to be driving most of tomorrow, just fyi if I don't respond." This is similar to the role that away messages play in many professionals' email inboxes: communicating to clients that any lack of response or delayed response is not due to a lack of respect, care, or professionalism but is instead a foreseen possibility. In a related vein, an individual can communicate a degree of respect and caring by timing messages that respect the recipient's schedule, such as by texting during business hours instead of at bedtime (Kayany et al., 1996).

Conversely, waiting an extended period of time before responding, or not responding at all, can make the recipient feel snubbed or forgotten. An example of intentionally communicating lack of PR is leaving a communication partner "on read," meaning that the partner knows that their message was received via electronic read receipt but is left unanswered for a significant duration. However, this slighting can also occur without intent, such as when a text or email is left unanswered by accident for days or weeks. A particularly egregious example of lack of PR is the practice of ghosting, or "the digital dissolution disappearance strategy" (LeFebvre et al., 2019). As we noted earlier in this chapter, individuals who are ghosted often do not receive communication that the relationship with the conversation partner is over but rather are left to interpret ongoing silence and lack of communication as signifying the end of the relationship.

Given the primary focus of this book, we provide an example here of ghosting in the context of psychotherapy rather than one that occurs in romantic relationships. This real-life example, with some identifying information concealed, was provided by a student in my (BAF) research lab studying PR:

> It was my first experience with a therapist and I sought therapy to deal with a trauma that I had previously never discussed with a professional. I wanted to be sure I was seeing someone qualified so I did extensive research and decided to spend a little more money than I initially planned because the therapist seemed like a good fit with my needs. I began with once weekly sessions, but after 2 weeks my therapist suggested we meet twice weekly. After attending therapy twice a week for 2 months, I felt my therapist knew a great deal about me.
>
> I had no school for an entire month over the winter holidays, so we decided that we would take a break while we were both away on vacation and resume when I returned to the city for my spring semester. About a week before returning I emailed her with an insurance question and a request to schedule our next appointment. A week went by and she never responded, so I forwarded her my initial email, assuming she just missed it and was catching up from being

away. Another week passed by, so I emailed her a third time. She immediately responded to this email, however only answering my insurance question and not to my request to restart our in-person sessions. I assumed it had to be a misunderstanding so I left her a voicemail, to which she never responded. At that point I was too embarrassed to continue attempting to contact her. We never had a tense moment or any difficulties between us, so I was extremely confused why she had dodged my every attempt at scheduling our next session. It almost made it worse that she responded to my insurance question because it confirmed she was reading my emails. It has now been over a year and I still have not heard from her.

The quick addendum here is that the research team was quite puzzled and intrigued by this event, one illustrating the antithesis of PR. We assumed that this therapist's actions constituted a remarkably rare phenomenon. However, the student who provided this example posted a question on Instagram, asking whether anyone knew of any similar incidents. Within a few weeks, dozens of people sent descriptions of how their own therapists had ghosted them (McMullen & Ort, 2021).

But to return to the ways in which PR can be demonstrated through social media: Another indication of engagement through private messaging is the length of one's message. Messages like "LOL," "Oh no!" or "OK" can be typed quickly but, in response to longer messages or emotionally vulnerable messages, can feel insubstantial and make the recipient feel unworthy of the sender's attention. Individuals can attempt to convey increased levels of care and warmth by writing longer messages and, as in FtF conversation, demonstrate a desire to continue speaking by asking follow-up questions. Asking questions is actually a more common tactic in text-only CMC than in FtF conversations (Antheunis et al., 2012), perhaps due to the lack of cues in CMC, such as not being able to see where one's conversation partner is physically located. By asking more questions of a conversation partner in text-based dyadic CMC, the partner is prone to not only disclose more but also feel increased closeness to the partner, likely as a result of feeling attended to.

O'Sullivan et al. (2004) used the term "politeness" to mean "following etiquette" and making "word choices" that communicate respect and courtesy. Much CMC is based on written exchanges (although video- and image-based CMC have become far more common with apps such as Instagram and Snapchat). Specific word choices may go a long way in the communication of PR from one participant to another, especially since individuals using CMC usually have more time to reflect on and choose their words than they do in FtF situations, and the recipients are aware of this. Word choices in CMC may go beyond expressing politeness in close relationships; researchers have highlighted the relational impact of positively and negatively valenced emotion words in instant messaging. For example, Slatcher et al. (2008) showed that explicit expressions of positive feelings toward another person in instant messaging predicted more relationship satisfaction for both the sender and recipient, as did sarcastic use of negative expressions of emotion. "Ugh, I *hate* you ;)" and "I love you so much" may both relay feelings of warmth and value to the recipient (the semicolon followed by a right parenthesis in this first phrase indicates a happy, winking face).

In addition to word choices, there are a variety of tools available to users of text-based CMC to communicate the warmth and affirmative stance emblematic of PR, including text-based nonverbal cues such as italics, bolding, asterisks, ALL-CAPS, and, especially, emoticons and emojis (Baym, 2010).

Most moderately tech-savvy individuals are familiar by now with emoticons and emojis. Both can be used to enhance the emotional tone of one's online messages; they can also be used to express or intensify negative emotions. Emoticons ("emotion icons") are characters on the keyboard—punctuation marks, letters, and numbers—used to create icons that represent specific emotions (e.g., happiness). Emojis are pictographs of faces, other body parts, objects, and symbols that may also be used to represent or intensify a response to another; the most common of these is the smiley face, usually intended to convey warmth or joy. Emoticons and emojis allow for nontextual cues analogous to facial and body language to be communicated in the instant-message context. Emoticons and emojis seem to allow for communication initiators to more explicitly emphasize parts of their message or to communicate more nuanced messages (e.g., sarcasm, tone), but their effectiveness in doing so remains open to debate. Derks et al.'s (2008) study suggested that emoticons that clash with the verbal component of CMC do not have sufficient ability to change the emotional verbal elements of the message. However, effective use of emoticons could support the provision of PR by helping to communicate warmth, informality, or humor.

In addition, written-out physicality (e.g., "giving you a hug"), GIFs (graphics interchange format) in the form of animations or video footage, and static images (e.g., pictures, cartoons, memes) all provide means of more clearly communicating tone and emotion than only text-based messages. While not always conveying positive emotions, they do demonstrate the sender's commitment to giving the recipient more emotional context to work with, often reflecting consideration for the recipient's emotional well-being. Note the difference, for example, between someone sending a text reading "IDK" versus sending an image (a meme, in this case) of a confused-looking man with the words "I don't know" at the top and the words "And at this point, I'm too afraid to ask" at the bottom. There are some indications (e.g., Pancani et al., 2021) that these phenomena are merely more technologically complex iterations of familiar interpersonal and social processes that figure prominently in our day-to-day lives. Still, digital natives continue to innovate ways to infuse semantic meaning, affect, and, inevitably, forms of PR into ever-evolving forms of CMC.

To summarize: The world outside of psychotherapy can provide therapists with new ideas about conveying PR. The way that Fred Rogers looked for the good in others and valued difference can, as noted earlier, inspire therapists to do the same. Therapists might also consult their own personal relationships for guidance, reflecting on when and with whom they felt most and least positively regarded: We suspect their findings will closely approximate those of the graduate students we consulted. According to these students, PR is most felt in relationships where consistency, genuine focused attention, and open acceptance are palpable and where judgment and implications of conditionality have no place. Finally, there is much to learn about PR from the world of social media. Therapists should be aware that however they decide to use CMC, the timing, length, and choice of words for their message(s) may all feel like meaningful reflections of PR, especially to clients who are digital natives.

We hope this journey along the road of PR, from Mister Rogers to contemporary social media, has helped elucidate the ubiquitous relevance of this quality in our day-to-day lives. PR is both a therapeutic common factor and a critical ingredient in a variety of extratherapeutic contexts, and these two settings have, over time, reciprocally informed one another. As therapists, remaining alert to the ways in which PR plays out in the ever-changing world around us is instrumental to understanding our clients' needs and expectations, as well as the complex connections we form with our clients.

As for Exhibit 5.1 earlier in the chapter, with quotes from Fred Rogers and Carl Rogers: All but the last quote was from Fred Rogers.

In the next chapter, we examine clients' perceptions of the nature and consequences of their therapists' PR—the perceptions that, according to Carl Rogers, count the most.

6

POSITIVE REGARD

Clients' Perspectives

No I won't be afraid . . . just as long as you stand, stand by me

–Ben E. King, "Stand by Me"

If asked what Carl Rogers considered the necessary and sufficient conditions for therapeutic change, most students of psychotherapy would likely list the therapist's positive regard (PR), empathy, and genuineness. While this answer is not exactly wrong—indeed, it's the answer Rogers himself often provided when summarizing his clinical theory in his filmed interviews—it's also not exactly right, either. It is an incomplete answer. As we noted earlier, in his 1957 paper, Rogers included several other, often-overlooked conditions. Most saliently, he contended that the therapist's actions and attitudes, regardless of how seemingly reflective they were of the three core therapist-provided qualities, would not make a difference until and unless the client experienced them. The client's subjective experience was paramount. In fact, Rogers (1951) had come to this conclusion some years before:

> It has become increasingly evident that the probability of therapeutic move-
> ment . . . depends primarily not upon the counselor's personality, nor upon

https://doi.org/10.1037/0000312-007

Understanding and Enhancing Positive Regard in Psychotherapy: Carl Rogers and Beyond,
by B. A. Farber, J. Y. Suzuki, and D. Ort

his techniques, nor even upon his attitudes, but upon the way all these are experienced by the client in the relationship. (p. 65)

However, because Rogers preferred thinking about PR as an overall attitude of acceptance and caring rather than comprising discrete interventions or "techniques" (a word he disliked when used as an indicator of his therapeutic style), he never really described what therapists actually *do* to engender the sense in clients that they are positively regarded. The consensus among his followers (e.g., Bozarth, 2001; Brodley & Schneider, 2001; Wilkins, 2000/2001) is that, for the most part, PR is manifest in the clinician's empathy. However, even if that is correct, it leaves open the question of whether there are ways in which PR may be demonstrated other than through empathy. The resulting ambiguity about what constitutes PR has left a regrettable, if somewhat understandable, void. It's difficult to discuss any significant aspect of therapy without some consensus or empirical basis for defining its properties or domain.

Several studies within the PR lab at Teachers College (Columbia University) have attempted to glean an understanding of the ways in which clients experience the nature and effects of therapist-provided PR. Among other questions posed by our research team: What kinds of therapist statements or actions do clients generally experience as positively regarding? Which therapist statements or actions demonstrating PR do clients perceive as occurring most frequently during the course of their therapy? Do clients believe there are optimal levels of therapist-provided PR? What do clients see as the impact of therapist-provided PR on the course and outcome of their psychotherapy? To what extent do identity considerations such as race and gender (of the client, the therapist, or both) play a role in the client's experience of PR? And last, how does engaging in teletherapy affect clients' perceptions of PR? In an attempt to gauge both an overall and an in-depth understanding of how clients view PR, these investigations have included quantitative (survey-based) research as well as qualitative (interview) studies. In this chapter, we review the results of these studies, with the hope that therapists gain a broad understanding of these issues from a client perspective in a way that may inform their clinical decision making.

In one such study (Suzuki & Farber, 2016), we recruited 540 psychotherapy clients, essentially evenly balanced between those who were currently in treatment ($n = 271$) and those who had terminated treatment ($n = 269$). The sample was primarily female (81.2%), White (79.1%), heterosexual (75.6%), and U.S. residents (83%); participants were, on average, 36.6 years old. Overall, the mean duration of therapy with the respondent's current therapist—or, among those who had terminated treatment, their most recent therapist—was just over

3 years (38.6 months). Therapy was conducted primarily in private-practice settings (66%), with therapists (according to respondents) practicing cognitive behavioral (43%), eclectic (20%), psychodynamic (13%), and humanistic–existential therapies (7%); 18% of the sample reported "other/not sure" for the type of therapy they were receiving. These therapists, according to respondents, were primarily White (83%) and female (70%).

We asked respondents to evaluate a series of interventions their therapist might engage in—statements and other actions that we hypothesized would reflect a positively regarding attitude. Initially, we compiled 60 possible items by reviewing the literature on PR, including the various statements by Rogers and other person-centered theorists (see Chapters 1 and 3) and the composition of already-existing surveys that assess PR (e.g., the Barrett-Lennard Relationship Inventory [BLRI]; Barrett-Lennard, 1964). This was a somewhat challenging task because the great majority of this literature, including assessment measures, steadfastly treats PR as an attitude rather than comprising discrete and/or observable actions. Furthermore, the standard measures of PR prioritize the acceptance aspect of PR to the relative exclusion of the more affirming/warmth/prizing aspect of this quality. In contrast, we chose to define PR in terms of "affirmation," privileging this aspect of PR.

We purposely included a wide variety of therapist comments, actions, and nonverbal conduct that, while not specifically identified in the person-centered literature as indicative of PR, might nonetheless be received by clients as positively regarding. We wanted to cast as wide a net as possible, without preconceptions, to see which therapist behaviors resonated with clients as having a high potential for PR—specifically affirmation. Thus, items included therapists praising clients for how hard they have been working in therapy, complimenting clients on a strength they possess, speaking in a gentle tone of voice, laughing at a funny comment a client has made, accurately summarizing what a client has said, stating that the client has handled a situation well, remembering the name or the details of someone or something clients spoke of long ago, allowing a session to continue overtime for a few extra minutes, maintaining good eye contact, smiling at a client, and hugging a client. The measure was iteratively refined through a series of pilot studies and by considering feedback offered by therapy clients and doctoral-level clinical psychology students.

Ultimately, 43 items were retained as a measure (Psychotherapist Expressions of Positive Regard [PEPR]; Suzuki & Farber, 2016) that was administered to our respondents as two separate but identical scales, each comprising 28 actions and 15 statements that therapists might use to demonstrate their PR. One scale, PEPR-Affirming (PEPR-A), assesses clients' perceptions of how affirming each of these statements and actions feels to them; the other, PEPR-Likely (PEPR-L), assesses their perceptions of the likelihood of these therapist actions and statements in their therapy. Both scales employ a 5-point Likert-type scale (1 = *not at all*, 3 = *moderately*, 5 = *to a great extent*).

WHAT KINDS OF THERAPIST STATEMENTS OR ACTIONS DO CLIENTS EXPERIENCE AS POSITIVELY REGARDING?

The therapist actions or statements that clients in this study viewed as most affirming—that is, those that garnered the highest average ratings on the PEPR-A scale—were quite thematically diverse, including promotion of client self-acceptance ("My therapist offers me a new way of understanding a part of myself that I usually view as a weakness"), nonverbal indications of active listening ("My therapist shows s/he is listening through her/his body language"), and even facilitation of insight ("My therapist makes a connection between my current experience and something I have discussed in the past"). Table 6.1 shows this survey's top 10 items that clients perceived as most affirming in their therapy.

What is arguably most significant here is the wide range of therapist actions that this heterogeneous group of clients perceived as most positively

TABLE 6.1. Clients' Perceptions of the Most Affirming (Positively Regarding) Therapist Actions

Item	M	SD
My therapist offers me a new way of understanding a part of myself that I usually view as a weakness.	4.30	.92
My therapist shows s/he is listening through her/his body language.	4.26	.93
My therapist makes a connection between my current experience and something I have discussed in the past.	4.26	.98
My therapist summarizes what I have said accurately.	4.25	.98
My therapist is understanding if I need to cancel or reschedule.	4.25	.98
My therapist remembers the name or the details of someone or something I spoke of long ago.	4.24	.97
My therapist maintains eye contact with me.	4.20	.99
My therapist compliments me on something I feel is a strength of mine.	4.19	.96
My therapist encourages me to take pride in the things I do well.	4.19	.95
My therapist speaks to me in a gentle tone of voice.	4.17	1.00

Note. Mean scores reflect scoring on a 5-point Likert-type scale wherein 1 = *not at all*; 3 = *moderately*; 5 = *to a great extent*. From "Toward Greater Specificity of the Concept of Positive Regard," by J. S. Suzuki and B. A. Farber, 2016, *Person-Centered & Experiential Psychotherapies, 15*(4), p. 272 (https://doi.org/10.1080/14779757.2016.1204941). Copyright 2016 by Taylor & Francis. Adapted with permission.

regarding (in terms of affirming qualities). In fact, most of these highly ranked items do not seem to fit into the paradigm for PR that Rogers and his followers laid out. The top-rated item, for example, "My therapist offers me a new way of understanding a part of myself that I usually view as a weakness," seems antithetical to a nondirective approach. Rather than acceptance or simple acknowledgment of a person's self-perceived weakness—actions that person-centered therapists hypothesize would ultimately lead to the client's greater self-acceptance—this action, of a therapist offering a client a new way of understanding this self-perception, is pointedly directive. And yet, it is an action that this sample of clients believed was quite affirming. Here is an excellent example of this kind of positively regarding behavior, one taken from the recent best-selling book *There There: A Novel* by Tommy Orange (2018). One of the protagonists, someone born with fetal alcohol syndrome (FAS), was speaking with his counselor:

> Karen tells me I don't have to worry about intelligence. She said people with FAS are on a spectrum, have a wide range of intelligences, that the intelligence test is biased, and that I got strong intuition and street smarts, that I'm smart where it counts, which I already knew, but when she told me it felt good, like I didn't really know it until she said it like that. (p. 17)

Much the same can be said of the third most highly ranked item here, "My therapist makes a connection between my current experience and something I have discussed in the past." Like the item noted in the previous paragraph, this item is far more consistent with the tenets of a psychodynamic approach and clearly extends beyond the act of acceptance. It suggests that demonstrating an understanding of a client or helping a client forge a greater understanding of themself may be a component of perceived PR, one that is distinct from (and more active than) acceptance and nonjudgement. More generally, it affirms the hypothesis that PR can be demonstrated through a diverse set of therapist-initiated actions, a finding that we see (later in this chapter) confirmed by interviews with clients.

Other highly rated items are more consistent with a Rogerian perspective on PR. Respondents on this survey indicated that they experienced high degrees of affirmation when their therapists listened attentively (e.g., "My therapist summarizes what I have said accurately," "My therapist remembers the name or the details of someone or something I spoke of long ago") and when therapists provided specific nonverbal or prosodic cues (e.g., "My therapist maintains eye contact with me," "My therapist speaks to me in a gentle tone of voice," "My therapist smiles at me"). Here is a fine example of nonverbal acceptance offered by a therapist, described by his client:

> 'Do you know what the most amazing thing was last week? I said, "I am incredibly needy" and you just raised your left eyebrow and held the palms of your

hands out and what you were saying was "so?" And actually, I went away from that session thinking: "I am very needy. So? What's wrong with that?" And I really experienced the acceptance in a non-verbal way that enabled me to accept my own fallibility. (Casemore & Tudway, 2012, p. 144)

To summarize: Whereas "positive regard" can be defined from a person-centered perspective as an attitude of acceptance, caring, or support, there are, according to clients, multiple ways for a therapist to demonstrate these attitudes. Furthermore, these actions are not exclusive to the tenets of person-centered or other humanistic therapies. These respondents are, in effect, stating that regardless of the type of therapy they are participating in, there is a wide variety of common therapist behaviors—both attitudes and interventions that have made their homes in treatment modalities outside of the person-centered community—that have the effect of making them feel positively regarded. From another perspective, these results suggest that therapists embracing multiple brands of psychotherapy are clearly willing and able to act in ways that effectively communicate PR to their clients.

WHAT KINDS OF POSITIVELY REGARDING STATEMENTS OR ACTIONS DO CLIENTS PERCEIVE AS OCCURRING MOST OFTEN IN THEIR THERAPY?

Again, the range of responses for clients' ratings of the most commonly experienced types of PR was extensive (see Table 6.2). This was, essentially, because there was great overlap between the top 10 most highly rated PEPR items for affirming quality and the top 10 items for likelihood of occurrence. Nine of the top 10 PEPR-L items also appeared in the top 10 PEPR-A list. This convergence can be seen as good news, suggesting that for the most part, therapy clients seem to find highly affirming those PR-like interventions their therapists most frequently offer. Although the limitations of self-report methods mean that findings like these are subject to client biases in recall, Rogers might redirect us to the tenet that the client's experience of the intervention, rather than the therapist's intervention itself, is most critical. Thus, that clients in our sample perceived that their therapists most frequently offered the interventions with the greatest power to convey PR is potent in itself, even if the objective frequencies are unverified.

One moderate exception to this finding is the item "My therapist offers a new way of understanding something that I perceive as a weakness." Whereas it was ranked highest (mean score of 4.30) in terms of its affirming potential on the PEPR-A scale, it barely qualified for inclusion in the top-ranked PEPR-L

TABLE 6.2. Clients' Perceptions of the Most Frequently Occurring Affirming (Positively Regarding) Therapist Actions

Item	M	SD
My therapist maintains eye contact with me.	4.31	.94
My therapist speaks to me in a gentle tone of voice.	4.27	1.00
My therapist is understanding if I need to cancel or reschedule.	4.11	1.16
My therapist shows s/he is listening through her/his body language.	3.99	.98
My therapist encourages me to take pride in the things I do well.	3.95	1.20
My therapist summarizes what I have said accurately.	3.86	1.14
My therapist compliments me on something I feel is a strength of mine.	3.85	1.18
My therapist makes a connection between my current experience and something I have discussed in the past.	3.85	1.23
My therapist remembers the name or the details of someone or something I spoke of long ago.	3.72	1.18
My therapist smiles at me.	3.71	1.08
My therapist laughs at a funny comment I make.	3.71	1.17
My therapist offers me a new way of understanding a part of myself that I usually view as a weakness.	3.71	1.18

Note. Mean scores reflect scoring on a 5-point Likert-type scale wherein 1 = *not at all*; 3 = *moderately*; 5 = *to a great extent*. From "Toward Greater Specificity of the Concept of Positive Regard," by J. S. Suzuki and B. A. Farber, 2016, *Person-Centered & Experiential Psychotherapies*, 15(4), p. 272 (https://doi.org/10.1080/14779757.2016.1204941). Copyright 2016 by Taylor & Francis. Adapted with permission.

item list, as part of a three-way tie for the 11th-place rank (Mean score of 3.71). This difference, while somewhat small in the context of a ranking of 43 items, is nonetheless significant for clinicians looking to enhance their clients' experience of PR. This is an intervention far more reflective of a cognitive behavior therapy or narrative approach to psychotherapy than it is of a person-centered therapist. Although pointedly directive, this action offers something therapy clients seem to hunger for: a compassionate way of understanding and accepting themselves. Whereas the respondents in our sample indicated that such interventions are by no means unheard of, their pattern of responses also implied that therapists might give some thought to how readily they reach for this particular clinical option, as their clients likely would not object to receiving more of it from them.

A comparison among the three items that address client strengths and weaknesses is also illuminating. The two items that focus on client strengths ("My therapist encourages me to take pride in the things I do well," "My therapist compliments me on something I feel is a strength of mine") are perceived as more common in therapy (Ranks 5 and 7, respectively), whereas the intervention perceived as most affirming of all the interventions queried—helping the client to reappraise a weakness—is perceived as less common (Rank 11

[tied]). Clients, it would seem, would prefer that their therapists affirm them by focusing not on their strengths but on the issues about which they feel vulnerable—yet they feel that their therapists are inclined toward the reverse. Being able to hold in equal esteem a client's strengths and weaknesses, rather than a positive bias toward emphasizing strengths, is vintage Rogers. A moving example of the power of a therapist's affirmation was posted by a client on the internet: "Whenever my therapist says she's proud of me I lose a year's worth of trauma" (Bologna, 2019).

Beyond the diversity of the list, another trend is notable: The most common interventions seem to be heavily weighted on the side of nonverbal signaling. Three of the top four most highly rated items were along these lines ("My therapist makes eye contact with me," "My therapist speaks in a gentle tone of voice," "My therapist shows s/he is listening with her/his body language"). Arguably, verbal indications of PR vary more significantly across treatment dyads than do nonverbal indications; that is, facial expressions and body language seem to be more universal modes of expressing PR than are verbal statements indicative of PR. A wise song lyric from "Wooden Ships" by Jefferson Airplane (1969): "If you smile at me, I will understand, 'cause that is something everybody everywhere does in the same language."

WHAT ARE THE CLUSTERS OF THERAPIST BEHAVIORS AND STATEMENTS THAT CONSTITUTE POSITIVE REGARD?

Several significant findings also emerged when the data of this study were subjected to a *factor analysis*, a statistical technique used to determine which item ratings cluster together and might therefore compose a unitary factor or distinctive component of PR. Three factors emerged. The first factor, which was significantly correlated with client ratings of the working alliance, we titled Supportive and Caring Statements. It consists of 15 hypothetical therapist *statements*, with the most representative items being "I'm glad you shared that with me," "This is a space for your own healing and growth," and "That must have been very difficult." This factor, then, is reflective of the way that most therapists and clients imagine PR being provided—essentially as therapist validation and/or affirmation. Imagine the following:

> Jordana has been seeing her therapist for a few weeks after struggling alone with months of low mood and overall life dissatisfaction. She has had trouble with fatigue and concentration, which are contributing to an overall feeling of inadequacy and stress at work. Parenting her toddler son has become increasingly difficult, as he has struggled with some behavioral issues at home, and she frequently finds herself snapping at him. Perhaps most challenging, her elderly

mother is in the early stages of dementia and is denying her diagnosis. Jordana, as the eldest daughter in her family of origin, has been trying without success to arrange in-home care for her mother, while her mother and her younger siblings insist this is unnecessary.

After Jordana has spent her first few sessions elaborating on her pervasive feelings of overwhelm and insufficiency, the therapist capitalizes on a momentary lull in the session. "Forgive me for saying so, but based on everything you're telling me, it seems as though you expect yourself to have superhuman capabilities. With everything you're struggling to digest about your mother's diagnosis and care, not to mention the demands of full-time work and parenting a young child, you somehow believe that you should be perfectly cheerful, efficient, and energetic in every moment, as well as a master negotiator ready to wear down the resistances of your own mother and siblings in the blink of an eye." Jordana begins to protest, and he asks her to let him finish: "From what I can see, it's clear to me that you are handling this difficult situation as well as anyone possibly can." Jordana, her mouth still open and ready to resume her stream of self-directed invective, begins to feel the full weight of his affirmation of her suffering and her efforts. This shift allows her to begin to transition from a posture of depressed self-recrimination toward a full allowance of her grief and terror, which she and her therapist then work together to process while generating a plan for how she can move forward to help herself and her family.

The second factor, Unique Responsiveness, was also significantly correlated with therapeutic alliance scores and consists of 11 therapist *actions* characterized by attentiveness and sensitivity to the patient's history and needs, with the three highest loading items being "My therapist summarizes what I have said accurately," "My therapist remembers the name/details of someone or something I have discussed in the past," and "My therapist offers me a new way of understanding a part of myself that I usually view as a weakness." These actions seem to reflect a particular attention to and respect for a client's individuality; most of these actions occur in multiple forms of psychotherapy. In fact, most of the items delineated within this factor are more often associated with psychodynamic therapy than with humanistic or other forms of psychotherapy. An example follows:

Keith has a history of manic episodes, some of which have landed him in the hospital in the last few decades. His associations to the experience of hospitalization are mostly negative—a parade of seemingly judgmental, white-coated clinicians, most of whom he sees once or twice and never again, very few of whom are interested in getting to know him. Yet, every so often, especially as he gets adjusted to his new medication regimen, he sometimes is able to have mutually satisfying exchanges with some of the other patients on the unit. Sitting in an art group with five or six other patients, he notices that the man next to him, his new roommate, has begun to shake and quietly whimper to himself. Keith recognizes that his roommate is clearly having some kind of flashback episode, the features of which the latter had confided in him the night before.

Keith reaches over to comfort his roommate, trying to remind him that he is safe, but the facilitator of the group mistakes this action for aggression, leading to an argument that is later written up in Keith's chart.

In discussing the incident with a social worker on the unit whom he has seen a few times and who visits him in his room after hearing what has happened, Keith dismisses the whole experience as a classic example of how he is always misunderstood and maligned by both the mental health system and other people in his life, as well as an example of racist attitudes that mistake even his most genuine efforts at showing care and compassion—since they come from a Black man—for aggression. The therapist listens attentively, draws parallels to Keith's early life experiences of trying to protect his younger brother from their abusive parents, and discloses to Keith that she is moved by his efforts at kindness and decency. After this session, Keith is surprised to feel understood and valued, in a way that begins to move the needle on his overall beliefs about mental health providers. He is astonished that his therapist, after meeting with him only a few times, has bothered to learn and recall details about his early history and is willing to see his perspective rather aligning herself as a monolith with the hospital staff.

Keith is even more touched when he later learns that the therapist has not only written an addendum in his chart clarifying the nature of the incident but also gone on record with her superiors to contest the inclusion of the incident report to begin with. As speaking out like this could have some workplace ramifications for her, it is truly an instance of the therapist's demonstrating "unique responsiveness" to Keith's history of discrimination, abuse, and systemic alienation. In a separate study (see the following), therapy clients like Keith articulated a therapist's willingness to go above and beyond the dictates of their role on behalf of the client as a clear indicator of PR.

Finally, the third factor that emerged from this study, Intimacy/Disclosure, includes six therapist *actions* representing extensions of the typical boundaries that exist in the therapeutic relationship, with the most characteristic items being "My therapist puts his/her hand on my shoulder," "My therapist hugs me," and "My therapist has tears in his/her eyes as I relate a sad story." These kinds of boundary-extending behaviors on the part of therapists can, on the one hand, feel quite affirming but can also, on the other hand, feel intrusive, nonprofessional, and even threatening. Indeed, for our sample, scores on the Intimacy/Disclosure factor were negatively correlated with ratings of the working alliance. The interventions of Keith's therapist in the preceding example—first, disclosing feeling personally moved by his kindness toward his roommate and openly sharing her own impressions of him as a caring and decent person and second, extending herself beyond typical boundaries by advocating on his behalf to her superiors—are examples of how therapists' actions within this domain may result in the client's feeling appreciated and positively regarded. Following is an example of how excessive extension of boundaries can result in the client's feeling overwhelmed and decidedly unappreciative of the therapist's actions:

> Camila, who seeks out a therapist for the first time, in response to long-standing difficulties with anxiety and occasional panic attacks, at first appreciates her therapist's informality, candor, and warmth. It feels like a sign of authenticity and closeness for her therapist to settle into the session by first asking how Camila is doing and then responding to Camila's polite reciprocation of the question by disclosing something that is going on with her—a tiff with her landlord or a childcare-related concern she is struggling with. Over the course of months, though, Camila notices that her polite inquiries have led to a pattern where increasingly large portions of the session are taken up with her therapist's personal concerns—a pattern that Camila has no idea how to get out of without seeming rude or inviting the hostility of her therapist. Camila is enacting a lifelong script of compulsive, excessive caretaking of others, to the exclusion of her own needs, and neither she nor her therapist seems able to name or challenge it. Eventually, Camila ghosts her therapist, feeling guilty but not knowing how else to proceed in a therapy that is clearly not helping her.

Subsequent analyses of these data focused on whether scores on these three factors are associated with clients' overall sense of being positively regarded (as per scores on the most common measure of PR, the BLRI). Consistent with our description of these factors previously, results showed that clients' sense that their therapists are being explicitly supportive and caring (Factor 1) and that their therapists are paying attention to them as unique individuals (Factor 2) are both associated with clients' overall sense of being positively regarded (per BLRI scores). The same, however, is not true of therapists' actions in the realm of self-disclosures and boundary extensions (Factor 3). What the analysis showed here was that clients' perceptions of these types of therapist actions are, in fact, negatively associated with their overall sense of their therapist's PR. It seems that for some clients, at least some of the time, these therapist behaviors can feel too intimate, even boundary crossing, thus detracting from a client's overall sense of being positively regarded.

The question of just how much a therapist should reveal to their clients has been hotly debated across the history of psychotherapy. As noted earlier, first-person accounts from Freud's analysands suggest that in practice, Freud was far more open, revealing, and interactive than his writings would indicate (e.g., Momigliano, 1987). Moreover, subsequent generations of theorists have persuasively disputed the notion that therapist neutrality is possible or even desirable, instead advancing a conception of therapy as an encounter that invariably involves self-disclosure on the part of both participants. Contemporary therapists across orientations generally agree that therapist self-disclosure should be used judiciously—it may even be more potent in lower doses—but that it can be helpful in modeling client disclosure and advancing treatment aims (Knox & Hill, 2003). We have more to say, later in this chapter, about self-disclosure and boundary extensions as helpful expressions of PR. But again, as noted previously, therapists need to be mindful of how reactive some clients can be to even well-intentioned actions, such as personal disclosures or a pat on the back. For clients who have been abused, for example, such boundary-extending behaviors can feel disrespectful or threatening—the antithesis of feeling positively regarded.

VARIABLES AFFECTING CLIENTS' PERCEPTIONS OF POSITIVE REGARD

Another aim of our research was to determine the extent to which variables such as client or therapist race, gender, or age, or characteristics of the treatment itself, are related to clients' experience of PR. Analyses of these data (Suzuki et al., 2019) indicated that although most of the variables studied did not have a significant association to clients' perceptions of PR, there were a few intriguing significant findings.

For example, self-identified LGBTQ respondents perceived Intimate/Disclosing interventions to be more affirming than did self-identified heterosexual respondents. For queer clients, an expression of intimacy or disclosure on the part of the therapist may serve as reassurance that the stigma their sexual identity can (unfortunately) carry in the broader society has no place in the treatment room. By contrast, international respondents, when compared with clients based in the United States, found Intimate/Disclosing interventions to be less indicative of PR, illustrating the importance of therapists' cultural sensitivity in considering how best to convey their caring for their clients. Further, non-White clients, in comparison with White clients, rated Supportive and Caring Statements as more positively regarding. The personal experiences of frequently marginalized and oppressed groups may prime them to be especially responsive to explicit expressions of PR.

We also found a significant negative association between client self-esteem and therapist provision of PR as reflected in scores on two of the factors: Supportive and Caring Statements and Unique Responsiveness. We interpreted this finding as evidence that therapists who perceive their clients as lacking in self-esteem make extra efforts to ameliorate these self-perceptions through these types of PR-related communications.

We found conflicting results for therapy type. When PR was measured using the BLRI—an instrument especially reflective of the concept of unconditionality (acceptance)—psychodynamic clients reported higher ratings of PR.

By contrast, when PR was assessed in our research via PEPR, a more multi-dimensional and behaviorally grounded instrument, cognitive behavior therapy clients reported higher ratings of PR on two of the three factors: Supportive and Caring Statements and Unique Responsiveness interventions. We hypothesize that while Rogerian principles have come to be incorporated into practice by clinicians of all stripes, infusing a degree of relatedness and warm acceptance into all therapeutic modalities, differing theoretical orientations have absorbed and implemented these ideas in divergent ways best suited to their underlying traditions (Farber, 2007).

Last, we found differences in treatment setting, with clients receiving therapy in outpatient hospital clinics and "other" settings reporting lower overall PR as compared with clients in private practice. This finding, further elaborated next, was replicated in the open-ended, qualitative study our team undertook next.

A QUALITATIVE STUDY OF CLIENTS' PERCEPTIONS OF POSITIVE REGARD

An additional study (Suzuki, 2018) was undertaken with a smaller number of participants to allow for a deeper and more nuanced exploration of the topic. Fifteen clients in a variety of psychotherapies were individually interviewed for approximately 1 hour and encouraged to reflect on their experiences with PR in therapy. We defined PR to these participants quite broadly—as "a feeling you get from your therapist that s/he likes you, accepts you, respects you, and/or has genuine interest in you" and as "a warm, caring feeling." Among other questions and prompts, respondents were asked to provide examples of situations in which they experienced PR, times when they experienced a lack of it, what they felt were the consequences of PR, and what they imagined therapists could do to better manifest this attitude. They were also asked to consider how the experience of PR might be affected by sociodemographic characteristics of both the client and the therapist. The data from these interviews were systematically reviewed, coded, and synthesized to produce domains, or major content areas. Although lacking in generalizability due to small sample size, the strength of qualitative research of this type lies in its richness and depth, allowing for a vivid picture of respondents' experiences.

The study results offer several key findings about PR in therapy, many of which confirm earlier clinical or empirical hypotheses: that PR is an essential ingredient in keeping clients engaged in therapy; that, in addition to facilitating the therapy process, it can promote growth and insight; that it can be communicated through a diverse range of therapist interventions; and that it has a close association with the facilitative conditions of empathy and congruence. These and other findings are explored in detail here. The qualitative study methodology (specifically, consensual qualitative research; Hill et al., 2005) allowed us to categorize how widespread a finding was within the sample using the following markers: A "general" finding signified that it had the endorsement of all or all but one participant in the sample, a "typical" finding meant that at least half of the participants had expressed the sentiment, and the "variant" label was applied to ideas that more than three but fewer than half of sample participants had expressed. Certain "rare" findings (two or three participants only) are also identified and discussed where salient.

Positive Regard as Fundamental and Impactful in a Healing Therapy Relationship

Almost without exception, study participants perceived PR as an active presence in their current therapy relationship and noted that the experience of PR increased over the course of their therapy. Participants described it as very important—in the words of one client, "a critical piece of my therapy."

To the extent that PR is an essential facilitative condition in therapy, how and what precisely might it facilitate? The general consensus was that PR strengthens the therapeutic relationship. All 15 respondents emphasized the role of PR in building a sense of ongoing connection and collaboration in therapy, highlighting the ways in which feelings of trust and safety are engendered by therapists' adoption of this attitude. One client recalled reacting to a striking display of PR from her therapist: "I thought, wow, she was committed to really being there in this relationship, and that meant a lot." In addition, therapist PR was commonly perceived to have a material impact on the therapeutic process. It was typical for participants to report greater ease with self-disclosure and self-exploration within therapy. As one participant explained,

> It makes it feel like I can say some of the irrational things I'm thinking or worrying about and not worry that I'm damaging my relationship with her because I know she likes me from the rapport we have built up.

Therapists' PR seemingly has the power to attenuate the shame and fear that can impede therapeutic progress and honest disclosure (e.g., Farber, Blanchard, & Love, 2019; Hill et al., 1993; Macdonald & Morley, 2001).

Participants also typically reported that PR buffers against therapeutic ruptures and keeps them coming back to therapy when they might otherwise decide to terminate. This finding is consistent with previous research indicating that the therapist's empathy and PR play a key role in retaining clients in treatment (Roos & Werbart, 2013). As one respondent in our study put it,

> Even if the session doesn't have a lot of progress in it, positive regard is maybe what keeps me in it. Like I walk away and think, "Well, it's still cool, I like talking to her and maybe we didn't make any progress today but in the grand scheme of things, our therapy relationship is still great."

This benefit of PR is particularly important during strains or ruptures in the therapeutic relationship. One client reflected on her response to a perceived slight from her therapist: "I had had six months of a foundation of positive regard, so I was able to address the issue. The foundation of positive regard helps me be clear and calm."

Another, related benefit of therapists' PR: More than half of our participants provided examples of how their therapists' PR increased their confidence in themselves and empowered them to make changes in their lives outside of therapy. One participant cited a change in her interpersonal functioning: "It's because of this support that I get that I'm able to feel good around other people. I'm not as needy as I was when I was younger." Another credited a positive career move to her experience of PR in therapy, saying, "I became a social worker because of my work with her. I built up my life again. And that's mainly because I've built up my trust of people through her trust in me."

Negative Consequences of the Lack of Positive Regard

Participants' recollections of experiences with a lack of PR further reinforced how essential they felt it to be in the treatment relationship. It was typical that clients could reference previous treatment contexts in which PR had been absent, with many of the participants stating that they had had one or more therapists in the past who conveyed PR rarely, if at all. Participants identified three consequences of experiencing a lack of PR in therapy. The first finding, with general frequency in the sample, was that a lack of PR caused the participant to feel upset or rejected. Respondents reported feelings including general discomfort and awkwardness, a sense of being "dismissed," "ignored," "frustrated," "invalidated," "fearful," "wounded," and "judged." A second, typical finding was that the lack of PR led to disengagement and, in some cases, to decisions to terminate. As one participant explained, "There's a sense of, 'why am I even talking to this person. They're gonna be dismissive. There's no place for what I'm saying to land.'" Another client recalled a previous therapist who rarely demonstrated PR: "I don't even remember what her face looks like because she didn't make enough eye contact with me, and I spent most of my time looking out the window." In short, a lack of PR is likely to result in therapeutic ruptures that lead clients to shut down, become less productive in therapy, and consider—or actually act on—terminating therapy.

Whereas a lack of PR had negative emotional consequences for the entire sample, a subset of clients attributed more severe consequences, such as intense and protracted emotional dysregulation and significant life disruptions, to a therapist's failure to provide PR. These participants reported that the negative feelings that accompanied the failure of a therapist to provide PR could compound their existing problems in ways that felt catastrophic to them. One participant stated, "I really tried to stick it out, but I got to the point that it was really making me worse instead of better." Although the particular presenting problems of the participants in the current study were unknown, their reports suggested that PR may feel like a lifeline that therapy clients who are particularly emotionally vulnerable cannot do without. Failure to adequately convey PR might therefore be considered among the foremost of therapist "treatment-destroying behaviors." That said, it's important to once again keep in mind that there are multiple ways for therapists to convey PR, and it may be difficult, especially in the early stages of a treatment, for therapists to be aware of which type is most important for specific clients.

What Does Positive Regard Look Like to Clients?

As it was a central question of the study, the interview encouraged participants to reflect, in great detail, on the instances in therapy in which they did and did not experience PR from therapists past and present. Not surprisingly, and consistent with Rogers's clinical practice, therapist *perspective taking*—essentially, conveying an empathic understanding of one's experience—was typically seen by participants as promoting PR. According to one participant, his therapist's willingness to "adopt the mystical language that corresponds to my inner world and imagination, and to really seem to get it" felt like a powerful demonstration of PR.

Another general response, and one consistent with our quantitative findings, was that therapists display PR through *nonverbal* means, via their body posture (leaning in), facial expressions (reflecting kindness), and tone of voice (gentle, calm). As one participant said, "I suspect that I don't experience as much positive regard when I'm on the phone with my therapist because I cannot see her face." Whereas most of the teletherapy being practiced during the coronavirus pandemic (circa 2020–2021) included face-to-face communication (via platforms such as Zoom or FaceTime), this respondent's statement underscores the need for studies to investigate the ways in which

PR's conveyance is influenced by the setting and medium of patient–therapist communication.

Similarly, the therapist's *warm and comfortable demeanor* was a typical signifier of PR, according to clients in this sample. Informality ("not being overly focused on paperwork or treatment planning"), frequent smiling, and use of humor were cited frequently within this theme. "She jokes with me, makes fun of me in a playful way," one participant explained. Another frequently cited and related theme was the therapist's *emotional engagement* in the therapy relationship, which included therapist attentiveness and presence during session, such as "keeping track of everything I have said from week to week." Emotional engagement was also indicated by a sense of mutuality in the therapy relationship, as when one therapist "asked for my input on her professional website design, showing she valued my opinion" or when another therapist said that "she was inspired by me, and she enjoys our conversations." These clients emphasized that they were engaged in a "real relationship" with their therapists, an idea that echoes Gelso's (2011) emphasis on the importance of this dynamic within the relationship and one that has considerable overlap with current conceptions of the salutary properties of therapist "presence" (S. M. Geller, 2013).

Yet another related and frequently cited theme: that therapist PR is often conveyed through *explicit affirmation, reassurance,* or *positive feedback.* According to one participant, her therapist's "stating directly that she likes and cares about me" is an effective way of communicating PR. Another said, "I was going through a tough time and was feeling very depressed, and I felt like my therapist was always encouraging; she was positive always. As I was putting myself down she would counteract that." This form of PR, as we've noted throughout these chapters, has been controversial for decades within the person-centered community. It's not what Rogers had in mind but seems to be what many clients (and therapists) accept and value as a legitimate aspect of this facilitative condition. The convergence between this qualitative finding and our earlier finding related to the facet of PR dubbed Supportive and Caring Statements lends further credence to this view.

In another general finding, the therapist's *authenticity and self-disclosure* were cited as common signifiers of PR in the therapy relationship. Instances of authenticity included the use of emotional self-disclosure and unflinching honesty—"telling it like it is without beating around the bush," as one participant put it. Other participants mentioned deriving a sense of PR from therapist communications that "show that he is human." Most participants who mentioned therapist self-disclosure specified the importance of context, in that the therapist's self-disclosures were experienced as positively regarding when they were "relevant to the therapy." Nevertheless, a few placed no such restrictions on the nature of therapist self-disclosure, deriving a strong sense of PR when they were privy to information about a therapist's life transition (e.g., having a baby, loss of a spouse) and were able to offer support to their therapist.

That authenticity and disclosure were cited so frequently and spontaneously by participants as clear manifestations of PR offers an important counterpoint to the mixed findings on the Intimacy/Disclosure construct from the quantitative study described earlier in this chapter. At least for the sample interviewed here, a sense of truly knowing who their therapist is and what he or she genuinely thinks and feels was prized above the need for strict boundaries or propriety, particularly as long as clients felt that the therapist's choices about disclosure remained grounded in the client's best interests. Of note, in a few cases, participants cited examples of boundary crossing (e.g., the therapist hiring the client as a babysitter, the therapist attending the client's wedding) as indications of PR. Here, as in the case of quite personal therapist disclosures noted previously, these instances can feel positively regarding due to the trust such boundary extensions imply. These instances are, however, relatively rare and seemingly seen by most clients (and therapists) as inappropriate, at least as likely to lead to therapeutic ruptures as they are to improved client functioning.

Relatedly, a few respondents spontaneously raised the issue of hugging their therapist—of whether being given implicit or explicit permission from their therapist to do so was a form of therapist PR. Although some clients who had hugged therapists either intermittently or regularly reported that this felt like an unequivocal and meaningful expression of PR, others (who might never have hugged their therapist) wondered whether it could or should have any place in the relationship. One client reflected, "It feels weird to have a close long-term relationship with someone where you absolutely can't touch them. And I can't ask because I'm too scared of rejection."

We hypothesize that the issue of physical touch may have confounded our negative findings for the Intimacy/Disclosure factor in our PEPR study, as the items that had particularly low PEPR-A scores were the ones that mentioned touching. While the experiences shared by participants in the current study under discussion suggest that hugging is by no means always a negative experience in therapy, it is clear that it is fraught. The wording of the PEPR-A items about touch—suggesting, as they did, unsolicited or even nonconsensual physical touch on the part of the therapist (e.g., "My therapist puts his/her hand on my shoulder")—may explain the contradiction in our findings on these two studies. We wonder if perhaps rephrasing the PEPR-A item from "My therapist hugs me" to "My therapist asks me if I would like a hug" may have accounted for the difference.

Two categories of therapist behavior that seem opposite in meaning were both seen as aspects of PR by respondents in this sample: *directiveness* on the one hand and *nondirectiveness and acceptance of feelings and experiences* on the other. Some participants reported that a therapist's active stance—for example, "gently helping me reorient to what I need when I get off track in session"—could serve to foster a feeling of PR. Another respondent said she enjoys the fact that she and her therapist can laugh together about many things but also that her therapist is "able to question when sometimes things aren't so funny; she acts as my conscience." Again, this aspect of PR, one that stands in contradiction to Rogers's and other person-centered therapists' belief in the necessity of therapist nonjudgment and nondirectiveness, is apparently an acceptable and appreciated PR-type offering according to some clients (and some contemporary person-centered theorists and therapists: see Chapter 3).

Conversely, many clients found an open, accepting stance toward whatever might arise in session to be crucial to their experience of PR, a clear vindication of Rogerian tenets. One participant who identified his therapy as "EMDR" (eye movement desensitization and reprocessing therapy) explained, "EMDR requires a lot of me, and some days I can't even get there but she's like, 'It's all okay.' She could say, 'You need to be concentrating more,' but she just starts over and says, 'Let's try again.'" Another reflected on her therapist's nondirective stance toward her past trauma: "My therapist provided positive regard by reassuring me that it didn't make me a bad person, but she also allowed me to get to my own truth, rather than her interpretation of what happened." It is noteworthy, too, that a majority of respondents voiced the sense that they experienced PR when their therapist was able to *create a balance between support and challenge*. Here, it seems, we are in the territory of what Stiles et al. (1998) referred to as "therapist responsiveness"—the ability to respond flexibly to the needs of clients.

Finally, participants typically saw the therapist's *flexibility around professional boundaries* as reflective of PR, a finding quite consistent with the results of the quantitative study noted earlier in this chapter. Indications of flexibility around boundaries included a relaxed approach to the therapeutic frame ("not being too strict about the session ending time"), availability over email, and willingness to reschedule if a client's circumstances dictated the need. One client reflected, "When she makes exceptions it shows that she is not trapped in her role." Some respondents also noted acts of advocacy and other significant gestures on their behalf. One respondent, for example, recalled that her therapist "on multiple occasions fought with my insurance company for better mental health coverage—she goes above and beyond."

Positive Regard: Can There Be Too Much of a Good Thing?

Can there be too much kindness or PR in life? Can it feel disingenuous if offered constantly? Shakespeare (1623/2003) seemed to think as much: "Yet I do fear thy nature; it is too full o' the milk of human kindness" (1.5.16–17).

In this qualitative study, we queried respondents as to whether they believed therapists could provide too much PR. Some answered in the hypothetical, as they themselves had never experienced an excess of this attitude: "I don't think I've ever felt too much, but I feel like too much might not be beneficial to the relationship. It would feel kinda false or not genuine. . . . You want to be positive but realistic." Respondents who had directly experienced the phenomenon reported a similar reaction: "I have had other therapists that I thought, 'Oh, get off it; you're being too gushy.' I've never felt that way from [my current therapist]. She's very mindful. . . . She doesn't say things just to say something." These clients seem to be implying that therapist genuineness can overlap with and catalyze client experiences of PR, a position supported by research indicating that these variables are significantly correlated (e.g., Gurman, 1977). Gurman (1977), in fact, suggested that genuineness is the core facilitative condition, a prerequisite for the provision of empathy and PR.

What Does a Lack of Positive Regard Look Like to Clients?

Participants were also asked to consider moments in therapy where they experienced a lack of PR, and the findings here often served as a mirror image of the behaviors described previously, though with less consensus within the sample. The most prevalent (and unsurprising) response, with typical frequency, was that *being unresponsive to the client, his or her needs, and his or her sensitivities* was experienced as a failure to show PR. Participants inferred unresponsiveness from a variety of therapist behaviors such as note-taking, appearing distracted, lack of communication regarding therapeutic boundaries, and lack of cultural sensitivity. As one participant noted: "My therapist suddenly decided to cut down the frequency of our sessions because she thought I was doing fine and she was out of town more frequently. But she never talked to me about it." Another participant offered the following example:

> The part of the country where I grew up, we talk slower, and my therapist is from a part of the country where they talk very fast, so I literally could not understand what she was saying. Whenever I asked her to slow down, she would for a little bit but then she'd go right back to the same pace.

Insufficient attunement to clients' experience is a potent signifier to clients that their therapists lack PR.

The second typically cited instance of lack of regard, somewhat related in nature, was therapist rigidity, either in terms of *rigid boundaries* or *rigid clinical structure*. This theme included therapist behavior related to self-disclosure. As one participant recalled,

> Once I asked my therapist if she was going to have another baby, and she was really caught off guard and just didn't want to answer me . . . it feels like I have to watch what I say to not make her uncomfortable.

Rigidity also emerged in terms of overly directive behavior from the therapist. One client recalled:

> My previous therapist was very structured and very homework driven. . . . If I came in and didn't have my homework done I really felt chastised, or if I was struggling in a certain area and really needed to talk about it, I could tell that she already had an agenda.

Other categories of therapist behavior were described by a smaller subset of participants as conveying a lack of PR. One variant finding was *combative* or *judgmental communication*, with several participants placing a premium on the tone of voice their therapists used: "I really felt barked at—the attitude and the feeling were accusatory. It was the complete opposite of feeling positive regard." Another theme noted by several participants—and, again, hardly a surprising one—was that *excessive boundary crossing* by the therapist could be experienced as a lack of PR. Most of the examples provided involved excessive disclosure of the therapist's personal information, such that "the relationship shifted to where I was listening to her problems. . . . And I was like, why am I paying you because we're talking about you." Some respondents specifically cited sexual themes as constituting the nature of the boundary violation. Clearly, it is imperative that in being open to providing PR through meaningful self-disclosures, therapists not lose sight of appropriate boundaries.

Identity Factors Influencing Client Perceptions of Positive Regard

Hoping to further elucidate the sociodemographic findings from our previous large-scale survey study, we invited participants in this interview to reflect on whether demographic or identity-related characteristics in themselves, in their therapists, or within the dyad had any bearing on their experience of PR. The specific characteristics of age, gender, sexual orientation, and race/ethnicity were included in the interview prompt, but participants mentioned a variety of characteristics when considering this question. For the most part, participants' views on which characteristics had relevance for PR were fairly idiosyncratic; however, a few broad generalities merit discussion.

Participants typically responded that they found it *easier to receive positive regard from a female rather than a male therapist*; this response was nearly universal in the sample. At least in part, this likely reflected a gender-match preference (13 of 15 participants in the sample were female); notably, though, both men in the sample also endorsed this theme. Other rationales for this sentiment included gender-role-based generalizations, such as the idea that "men are less calm, soothing, and compassionate" than women.

Some preferences emerged in the sample regarding the therapist's age. A typical theme was that an *older or more experienced counselor conveys positive regard more effectively* than a less experienced or younger counselor. Participants (mean age = 48) substantiated this impression by explaining that they had experienced more positive regard with older therapists in the past. While a few respondents were dismissive of younger or less experienced therapists without much explanation, one suggested that more experienced therapists were better able to be clinically flexible: "She has twenty years of experience . . . we were just able to do what I needed." However, a significant minority of participants expressed the sentiment that *age match with the therapist promotes positive regard*. These respondents stated that they felt more comfortable and better able to relate to their therapists if they were going through similar phases of life. One explained,

> When I turned 70, she was about to also, and we talked about that in a way that made it a little more personal than if she were just a more distant therapist who wouldn't acknowledge that we were the same age.

While some participants suggested that sexual orientation and race/ethnicity—either theirs or their therapist's—influenced their sense of receiving PR, this perspective was not widely shared. This finding runs somewhat counter to suggestions in the literature that PR may be particularly essential to work with clients from marginalized or stigmatized populations (e.g., Lemoire & Chen, 2005). One possibility is that social desirability concerns might have hindered respondents from voicing the idea that they would not relate as easily to a therapist of a different race, ethnicity, or sexual orientation.

Moreover, given that the vast majority of the therapeutic dyads described in the sample consisted of White clients (primarily female) with White therapists, the lack of positive findings here should be viewed with caution. These results may be best understood as capturing the perspectives of White female clients on the relevance of demographic factors for therapists' provision of PR. A separate study focusing on the experiences of racial and ethnic minority clients could offer more comprehensive results on the role of PR in racially mixed and matched therapist–client dyads, either confirming or providing alternative perspectives on the lack of association found, in this study, between race/ethnicity and clients' experiences with PR.

Furthermore, the majority of participants provided rich accounts of the extent to which dyadic demographic factors (including ones not specifically queried, such as socioeconomic background, marital status, and religion), as well as contextual factors, such as the setting in which therapy occurred (e.g., private practice vs. clinic or hospital), were particularly salient for their experience of PR. However, these data were idiosyncratic and could not be fit into coherent patterns in sufficient numbers to be captured by the research paradigm. One example, though, is that of a respondent who spoke of her lack of feeling positively regarded in working with a series of therapists within a hospital setting: "I would get changed on such a regular basis—once you got a connection with somebody, they were gone." This finding corroborates the result obtained in our earlier survey study, making the case that clinical setting is a significant and understudied factor in the provision of PR. Shorter courses of treatment, high caseloads, bureaucratic demands, and frequent clinician turnover found in understaffed or highly institutionalized settings might well lead to increased stress and burnout, while curtailing clinicians' ability to draw on the necessary inner resources to relate to clients with warmth, acceptance, and empathy. The overall picture here, though, is that each client comes to the therapy relationship with their own personally meaningful set of sociodemographic identities and is sensitive to similarities and differences within the dyad according to these priorities; this is the basis for multicultural counseling (e.g., Sue et al., 2019). There exist rich opportunities for the therapist–client dyad to explore these perspectives in a way that promotes PR.

Optimizing Positive Regard: Clients' Wish List

Participants were asked how their therapists might enhance or improve the experience of PR in therapy. With only a few exceptions, clients were largely satisfied with the PR offered by their current therapists and tended to respond to this question with some form of the advice "Do more of what you're already doing." But they did offer three suggestions for enhancing PR in significant enough numbers to be captured in the analysis. The first of these, occurring in more than half the sample, was to *be attentive and responsive to the client as an individual.* It was recommended that therapists signal that their clients have their undivided attention by being mindful of nonverbal cues and by asking questions and keeping the focus on the client. Therapists were also advised to display attentiveness and responsiveness by intervening in ways that reflected awareness of the client's individuality. One participant summarized this as follows: "Try to see each person uniquely. Don't try to peg them into categories. Focus on my strengths and what I can do, not what I can't do." Other participants felt that responsiveness could include attention to weaknesses as well: "I have strengths and weaknesses, and my therapist should help me compensate where I'm weak and congratulate me where I'm already strong."

A second theme, occurring in half the sample, was that therapists should *be transparent and communicative* with their clients, a response reflective again of the overlap between PR and genuineness. Respondents expressed the desire not to be left in the dark in a variety of contexts. One client said, "I don't really like the silent therapist because you just have no idea what they're thinking." Another added, "It would feel more like a human relationship if she gave me more of her feedback and insight." For others, the preference for open communication related to policies and the therapeutic frame. One participant, whose therapist was canceling sessions to go out of town with increasing frequency, said that she wished her therapist would explain the situation more: "It's like I'm not sure what's happening or what's going to happen. And I don't like having that feeling . . . I wish she would speak about it more." Another expressed a preference for greater clarity around the bounds of touch:

> I think that they should talk about it during the first couple sessions when they're talking about other rules like cancellation policies. I think they should just bring up touching. Like, "If you ever need a hug you can ask me, I'm open to hugging." Or, "I don't hug clients under any circumstances."

One final suggestion, also voiced by half the sample, was for therapists to *take a caring and nonjudgmental stance* in order to most effectively communicate PR. Here, of course, we're in the classic realm of PR as first articulated by Rogers. Respondents endorsing this theme highlighted the personal aspect of the therapy relationship, with one saying that "positive regard gives you the feeling that you are in the presence of your friend. Someone who cares about the outcome, who cares about you, and tries to take into account the broadest possible perspective." Along these lines, one client emphasized that a therapist's empathic, nonjudgmental stance was critical—"really trying to put yourself in their shoes and not to come across as judgmental."

Three Core Features of Positive Regard

To synthesize: The participants in this interview study catalogued multiple and diverse instances of therapist expressions of PR, suggesting that therapists have broad options when considering how best to express this attitude to their clients. Nonetheless, respondents' experiences of PR, wide-ranging though they were, seemed to cohere around a few core attitudes that offered a vivid picture of what PR—and its absence—looks and feels like to clients. Three recurrent thematic strands emerged, each of which consists of overlapping therapist attributes.

Cluster 1: Warm Authenticity

The first core feature of PR is that it is *experienced through a warm and authentic relationship with the therapist.* Respondents often spoke of warmth (e.g., explicit affirmation and a warm and comfortable demeanor). They also referred consistently to the role of therapist authenticity, often recollecting instances where they especially felt their therapists' emotional engagement and willingness to be self-disclosing. Thus, and as noted earlier, clients' experiences of PR seem inextricably connected with another facilitative condition— therapist congruence or genuineness. But deviating from classical client-centered thought, these respondents felt that this warmth/authenticity aspect of PR was manifest by their therapist's ability to provide explicit affirmation as well as to provide a balance between support and challenge.

However it is expressed, participants overwhelmingly agreed that the therapist's authenticity is what allows them to derive therapeutic benefit from PR. Whereas none of our respondents noted that authenticity and PR can be at odds when the therapist is expressing strong negative feelings toward a client, this situation has posed a dilemma for some person-centered theorists (Bozarth, 1998; Wilkins, 2000/2001). The partial solution to this problem lies in the therapist's ability to maintain a benign, caring attitude toward a client, even as the therapist is offering feedback that may be difficult for the client to hear. We have more to say about this issue in Chapter 8 inasmuch as one of the therapists featured in that chapter (Dr. Betsy Glaser) epitomizes the ways a wise therapist can negotiate these seemingly antithetical positions; we also return to this issue in greater detail in Chapter 9, when we review the controversies that have arisen around the definition and appropriate parameters of PR. However, the co-occurrence of warmth and authenticity in these interviews suggests that in the minds of most clients, PR and authenticity are typically synergistic.

Cluster 2: Flexible Responsiveness

The second cluster reveals that *flexibility and responsiveness to the client* are core markers of PR. Therapists' ability to flexibly accommodate and respond to the needs and concerns of clients was frequently cited as an indication of PR. Therapist responsiveness—for example, to client feedback—seems to act as a signal of PR because it indicates that their therapist truly values what they have to say and what they need. Responsiveness and flexibility also occur when therapists are willing to deviate from policies and standard practices as dictated by context or circumstance. Often, this involves flexibility around boundaries, such as being available over email or extending the session when a client arrives late or seems to be in crisis. In being clinically responsive and flexible, the therapist acknowledges the client's uniqueness and that one size does not fit all, further reinforcing the sense, discussed previously, that they are engaged in a real relationship and not merely a clinical transaction.

Of note, both the quantitative and the qualitative studies previously described identified responsiveness as a core feature of PR (the former with the dimension of "unique responsiveness" and the latter with the "flexible responsiveness" cluster), thereby strengthening the impression of its validity and relevance to PR. Though these are the first two studies to demonstrate a link between responsiveness and PR, Bohart (2015) suggested much the same in describing the evolution of his own clinical work (see Chapter 3, this volume). Responsiveness has been described by Stiles et al. (1998) as therapist behavior that is affected by emerging context. "Appropriate responsiveness" is the extent to which therapists' choice of treatments and interventions in a given moment is shaped by their attention and sensitivity to a client's verbal and nonverbal behavior.

This emphasis on therapist responsiveness aids in the interpretation of seemingly contradictory findings from our qualitative study—for example, the fact that both nondirectiveness and directiveness from the therapist were cited as markers of PR. For a certain client in a given moment, a therapist's provision of structure and authority may be experienced as particularly containing and nurturing, and feeling taken care of in this way may contribute to feeling positively regarded. In another moment or with a different client, a more receptive and flexible attitude, coupled with the sense that the therapist lacks a preconceived agenda, is more likely to lead to feeling accepted and cared for. Viewed in this way, the wide range of therapist behaviors that have been identified as markers of responsiveness can be better understood; context is key in inferring responsiveness. Responsive therapists are attuned to clients' reactions to these different approaches on a moment-by-moment basis and titrate their interventions accordingly; in so doing, they effectively communicate PR by letting clients know that their experience as individuals is of utmost importance.

Cluster 3: Empathic Acceptance

The third cluster of themes suggests that central to clients' experience of PR is a *therapist's attitude of empathic acceptance*—the ability to convey a deep understanding of clients' subjective experience. For many clients, the experience of being understood goes hand in hand with a sense of being accepted and positively regarded. Many participants were emphatic in conveying their sense that empathy and acceptance allowed them to feel safe to open up in therapy without fear of shame or judgment. Therapists' efforts to understand their clients' experiences reflect the regard in which they hold their clients; furthermore, genuine expressions of caring, affirmation, and acceptance are all the more potent in the context of feeling known and understood.

Taken together, our quantitative and qualitative explorations of PR converge on several key findings. Both studies support the idea that PR substantially facilitates the development and maintenance of the overall working alliance and that PR can be conveyed through multiple means, including specific therapist statements and actions. In both studies, we found indications of a three-factor structure. Though not identical, both of these tripartite structures featured the construct of therapist responsiveness as a core feature of PR. Finally, in both studies, we found support for the convergence of empathy and PR.

A few differences across the studies also bear noting. In our survey data, the Intimacy/Disclosure factor was negatively associated with an overall measure of PR (the BLRI); in our qualitative study, respondents spoke favorably of the value of their therapists' "warm authenticity." As discussed earlier, we believe that, taken together, these findings point to the distinction between an indiscriminate relaxation/violation of boundaries—especially physical ones— in the therapy relationship and a carefully considered extension of boundaries that is executed with attention to clinical need and context. With this in mind, the studies make a strong case that authenticity is also intertwined with the experience of PR, yielding an overall impression that the three facilitative conditions are usually interrelated aspects of the therapist's caring stance. Finally, these two sets of data offer somewhat inconsistent accounts of the client experience of PR through the lens of sociodemographic variables such as race, gender, and sexual orientation. Further investigations with larger and more diverse sample sizes are called for to more fully contextualize the findings here.

In summary, the two studies previously discussed confirm many of the assumptions of Rogers and his followers about the nature and functions of the therapist's provision of PR. But what clients also suggest is that Rogers omitted something significant from his work on PR: that this attitude can be conveyed through therapists' adoption of a flexible clinical style, one that may be at times directive and challenging, highly self-disclosing, explicitly complimentary, or even interpretive (e.g., offering clients new ways of understanding themselves). David Cain (2010), a colleague of Rogers and the founder and former editor of the *Person-Centered Review*, suggested much the same:

> Therapist acceptance, regard, and affirmation are sentiments that often need to be expressed tangibly to the client to have optimal therapeutic effect. Such

expressions may take many forms such as smiling, warm vocal tone, consistent eye contact, shared laughter, celebrating the client's triumphs, looking pleased to see the client, self-disclosure about something that the therapist values in the client . . . among many others. (p. 84)

In listening to the voices of therapy clients, it is clear that there are many reasons that clinicians might wish to optimize their clients' experience of PR. From the outset of therapy, clients are attuned to indications of PR in their therapists' behavior. Furthermore, a foundation of PR developed early in the relationship can pay substantial dividends later, as the therapeutic dyad works through particularly thorny issues that require high levels of client motivation, safety, and trust. Clients' voices clearly suggest the importance of therapists' working actively to convey warmth, respect, and interest—in a fashion authentic to their personal style and consistent with their theoretical leanings—from the start of treatment.

CLIENTS' PERCEPTIONS OF POSITIVE REGARD, TELETHERAPY, AND THE CORONAVIRUS PANDEMIC

We gained the opportunity to learn more from clients themselves about how they experienced PR under unprecedented circumstances when the coronavirus pandemic escalated rapidly in early 2020. Despite the fact that remote forms of psychotherapy have historically been viewed as less desirable by clients as well as therapists (and less reimbursable through insurance plans), most therapists had no choice, due to mitigation and social distancing measures, but to shift to teletherapy practice (i.e., psychotherapy online or over the phone). One question of interest, then, is how this transition has affected clients' engagement in treatment, including their perceptions of their therapists' ability to convey PR. Over 2 years later, this question is more relevant than ever, as the pandemic wears on and teletherapy appears to be here to stay as a standard treatment option. In hearing from clients who had made the transition during this period, we were able to understand how teletherapy can open new opportunities for clients to experience PR in treatment.

Therapists certainly face a number of obstacles when conducting teletherapy, including reduced opportunities to be attuned to clients' body language, increased fatigue related to working online and excessive screen time, and technological challenges and delays (Feijt et al., 2020; S. Geller, 2020; Nitzburg & Farber, 2019). Actions that clients might perceive as innocuous, or even facilitative, in traditional in-person therapy (e.g., taking notes) may be seen in online therapy as evidence of clinician lack of interest or distraction (Openshaw et al., 2012). In addition, the lack of the therapist's physical presence—the inability to hand that box of tissues to the client, the inability to move closer, the sense of not being in the same space—can attenuate the ability to be close to and supportive of one's client. Despite these challenges, nascent research supports the notion that a positive working alliance can be established through teletherapy, with reports of moderate to strong therapeutic alliance ratings across therapeutic orientations (e.g., S. Geller, 2020; Germain et al., 2010; Goldstein & Glueck, 2016; Simpson & Reid, 2014). Some research has also indicated that, post-termination, clients in teletherapy report experiencing high levels of empathy during their treatment (Openshaw et al., 2012).

Our large-scale study (N = 2,337) of clients' perceptions about transitioning to teletherapy as a result of the coronavirus pandemic (Ort & Farber, 2021) added to the impression that therapy clients are able to receive PR just as well—indeed, in some cases, even more strongly—within the teletherapy frame. As part of this study, respondents used a 5-point Likert-type scale (1 = *much less*, 3 = *about the same*, 5 = *much more*) to rate the extent to which their therapists' provision of specific expressions of PR has changed in the transition from in-person therapy to teletherapy. The results indicated that clients perceive their therapists to be as or more positively regarding in the context of teletherapy as in-person therapy. For example, slightly more than 93% of clients reported that their therapist was now about the same or more affirming, complimentary, friendly, warm, and empathic than they were before the shift to teletherapy. In addition, slightly more than 85% of this sample reported that, posttransition, their therapists are either as good at or better at making them feel cared about and appearing interested in what they have to say. It is notable, too, that on an item measuring client disclosure, nearly 75% of the clients in this sample reported that in their teletherapy sessions, they disclosed either about the same or even more personal material to their therapist than they had in-person. Although this change cannot be attributed solely to the perceived increase in PR from their therapists, some association is likely.

However, despite therapists' ability to effectively provide PR via teletherapy, only 54% of clients in this survey reported feeling about the same or more connected with their therapist; 47% reported feeling significantly less connected to their therapist during teletherapy. One explanation for this apparent paradox is that even as clients feel less connected to their therapists over teletherapy—the physical distance feels palpable to many—they are more aware of therapists' efforts to "close the gap" by being especially warm, friendly, and affirming. Perhaps, too, the tendency, during this pandemic, for both members of the therapeutic dyad to check in with each other regarding health and safety concerns has increased clients' perceptions of their therapist's caring, supportive, and accepting attitudes toward them. These findings suggest that it may be prudent for clinicians who are trying to communicate PR to be especially sensitive to how their actions, including their physicality, may be interpreted differently in teletherapy and to offer clarifying statements to their clients in order to avoid misunderstandings (e.g., "If you see me looking off to the bottom right here, it's because I'm taking notes on what you are saying").

In sum, PR remains largely preserved—and, in some ways, even enhanced—in the transition from in-person therapy to teletherapy. How might we understand this? Although some significant structural elements of therapy have changed in the transition to teletherapy, the basic elements of PR—the therapist's acceptance, care, support, and empathy—are all eminently conveyable through the most common currently practiced forms of teletherapy (i.e., those that include video features, such as FaceTime and Zoom). In addition, as noted earlier in this chapter, there are other, less intuitive aspects of therapist-provided PR that clients have identified, including therapists' ability to offer clients new ways of understanding themselves, therapists conveying active listening through body language, therapists making connections between clients' current and past experiences, therapists accurately summarizing clients' experiences, and therapists complimenting and taking pride in clients' achievements—all which are conveyable via teletherapy. Finally, although teletherapists are not physically present to clients, as they are in face-to-face therapy, they may have unique means to communicate PR, such as the locational flexibility to see a client during a family crisis that has taken the client out of town or, as in text therapy, the temporal flexibility to let a client take hours to respond to a difficult question. These departures from the traditional frame of psychotherapy can create treatment challenges, but they also provide new ways for clinicians to demonstrate care, support, and warmth for their clients.

In the next chapter, we consider therapists' perspectives on PR: what they see as constituting PR and how they view its importance and influence on therapeutic processes and outcomes.

7

POSITIVE REGARD

Therapists' Perspectives

Tell them that, to ease them of their griefs, their fears of hostile strokes, their aches, losses, their pangs of love, with other incident throes that nature's fragile vessel doth sustain in life's uncertain voyage, I will some kindness do them.

—William Shakespeare, Timon of Athens

Carl Rogers maintained that the client's subjective experience was paramount, that ultimately the only thing that "counted" was whether a client felt their therapist's empathy, genuineness, acceptance, and caring. As such, our lab's first foray into investigating the nature of positive regard (PR) was to study clients' perceptions of the ways in which their therapists most often conveyed PR and their perceptions of which of these ways felt most affirming. As Chapter 6 documented, clients construe a great variety of therapist statements and behaviors as highly positively regarding, many of which, like the therapist's offering a new way of understanding a client's perceived weakness, seem to be beyond the traditional bounds of person-centered psychotherapy.

https://doi.org/10.1037/0000312-008
Understanding and Enhancing Positive Regard in Psychotherapy: Carl Rogers and Beyond, by B. A. Farber, J. Y. Suzuki, and D. Ort

Nevertheless, we also thought it important to understand whether therapists' perceptions of providing PR were consonant with patients' sense of receiving it. Our belief in the value of this undertaking was also reinforced by the findings of a previous study: that therapists viewed their expressions of respect or admiration for clients as that form of self-disclosure that most advanced treatment aims (Lane et al., 2001). Thus, our research team designed a study (Farber & Ort, 2021) that tapped three broad areas: (a) therapists' assessment of the importance of PR in their practice, (b) therapists' sense of which specific aspects of PR they regard as most affirming and which of these aspects they most often provide to their clients, and (c) therapists' sense of whether and under what circumstances PR should be modified as a function of client identity-related factors.

Our sample comprised 269 licensed psychotherapists who were mostly female (80%), White (87%), heterosexual (88%), and residing in the United States (93%). On average, these participants were 40.5 years old ($SD = 15.17$). They included those with a PhD (33%), master's degree in psychology (32%), master's degree in social work (9%), and PsyD (12%). Their primary theoretical orientation included cognitive behavioral (27%), psychodynamic (22%), integrative (19%), other (18%), humanistic–existential (6%), dialectical behavior (4%), and interpersonal psychotherapy (4%) therapies. They had been seeing clients for an average of 13.57 years ($SD = 12.76$) and conducted their work in a variety of locations, including private practice (47%), community mental health (30%), student/university health (12%), and hospital outpatient (5%) settings.

These respondents completed a self-report measure (Psychotherapists' Perceptions of Positive Regard [PPPR]) that included both quantitative (survey) questions and qualitative (open-ended) questions.

PSYCHOTHERAPISTS' PERCEPTIONS OF THE ROLE OF POSITIVE REGARD IN TREATMENT PROCESS AND OUTCOME

One section of our PPPR measure was designed to investigate the extent to which therapists view PR as central to their clinical work, perceive the relative importance of several of its components, and envisage these components as important to their clients. This section also investigated the extent to which therapists consider PR as impactful in regard to the alliance, therapeutic ruptures, and treatment outcome. It includes 18 items (e.g., "To what extent does PR play a role in guiding the work that you do?") answered on a 5-point Likert-type scale ($1 = $ *not at all*, $3 = $ *moderately*, $5 = $ *to a great extent*).

Consistent with the views of Rogers, we defined PR to therapists in our study as anything they might do to convey interest, acceptance, respect, care, and a feeling of liking toward their clients. The mean score of the first question posed to our respondents, "To what extent does positive regard play a role in guiding the work that you do?" was 4.5 (*SD* =.70). From another metric: The great majority of the sample (90%) indicated that PR guided their clinical work *to a great extent*.

That a heterogeneous sample of therapists representing a range of theoretical orientations overwhelmingly acknowledged PR as central to their clinical work reflects an important historical shift. When Rogers (1957) first identified unconditional positive regard (UPR) as one of the "necessary and sufficient conditions" for therapeutic success, he faced considerable pushback from clinicians—psychoanalytic therapists rejected his noninterpretive approach, and behavioral therapists rejected his focus on clients' subjective feelings. Even when many Rogerian ideas became more mainstream during the latter part of the 20th century, as clinicians of virtually every variety accepted— and even touted—the importance of relational factors (Farber, 2007), many viewed the provision of PR and, even more so, UPR as unnecessary, unrealistic, or even inimical to client growth (see Chapter 9). But now, more than 6 decades after Rogers introduced the term in his writings and shorn of its exclusive association to Rogers and humanistic therapy, the results from this survey question suggest that nearly all therapists recognize PR (albeit not in its unconditional form) as a clinically significant aspect of their work.

Next, to understand which components of PR therapists regard as most important, we listed several that have been noted consistently in the literature (see Chapters 1 and 3) and asked respondents to rate how important each is to them in their practice and how important each might be to their clients.

As seen in Table 7.1, respondents in our study were particularly impressed with the extent to which five of these six listed components constitute significant aspects of their provision of PR. Respect, acceptance, empathy, care, and interest all garnered mean scores of 4.2 or higher on the 5-point scale. Four of these items were regarded by 90% or more of our respondents as important *to a great extent*; the other item, "interest," was deemed important *to a great extent* by over 80% of the sample. The outlier here was respondents' evaluation of the importance of liking their clients. "Liking" was not regarded as unimportant per se (*M* = 3.27, *SD* = 1.04) but rather considerably less important as a component of PR than the other elements listed.

As Table 7.2 indicates, therapists' evaluations of the importance of specific PR components to their clients closely approximates their own sense of the importance of these aspects. But there was one notable exception to this general trend: Therapists believed that their clients placed far greater importance on the need to be liked than they (therapists) believed it was important to like them (clients). In comparison with their tempered sense of

TABLE 7.1. Therapists' Perception of the Importance of Discrete Components of Positive Regard in Clinical Practice (*N* = 269)

Component	*M*	*SD*	*Not at all*	*Moderately*	*To a great extent*
Empathize with your clients	4.71	.60	1%	4%	95%
Care for your clients	4.70	.61	2%	2%	97%
Respect your clients	4.69	.67	1%	5%	94%
Accept your clients	4.59	.78	3%	8%	90%
Feel interested in your clients	4.24	.91	6%	13%	81%
Like your clients	3.27	1.04	24%	35%	42%

Note. Mean scores reflect scoring on a 5-point Likert-type scale wherein 1 = *not at all*; 3 = *moderately*; 5 = *to a great extent*. From *Therapists' attitudes regarding the communication of positive regard* [Paper presentation], by B. A. Farber and D. Ort, 2021, Society for Psychotherapy Research Annual Meeting. Copyright 2021 by B. A. Farber and D. Ort. Reprinted with permission.

how important it is to convey liking a client as part of the expression of PR, therapists indicated a belief that feeling liked was quite important to clients themselves (*M* = 4.40, *SD* = .77). Fewer than half (42%) of our respondents suggested that liking their clients was important *to a great extent*; in contrast, far more than half (87%) contended that clients' perceptions of feeling liked was *to a great extent* an important aspect of PR. This discrepancy touches on the intriguing question of whether PR needs to be genuine in order for clients to experience it as such. Rogers believed that the therapist needed to truly feel a sense of respect and acceptance toward the client in order to communicate real PR. So—what might be happening here?

Perhaps many therapists believe that their professional role requires them to at least occasionally feign liking their clients in order to further the course of therapy. As we noted previously (see Chapter 3), research has found that concealing feelings of frustration toward clients and falsely implying that

TABLE 7.2. Therapists' Perception of the Importance of Discrete Components of Positive Regard to Their Clients (*N* = 269)

Component	*M*	*SD*	*Not at all*	*Moderately*	*To a great extent*
Respect them	4.82	.47	0%	3%	97%
Accept them	4.80	.48	0%	3%	97%
Empathize with them	4.78	.51	.43%	3%	97%
Care for them	4.73	.57	0%	6%	94%
Feel interested in them	4.68	.60	.43%	6%	94%
Like them	4.40	.77	2%	11%	87%

Note. Mean scores reflect scoring on a 5-point Likert-type scale wherein 1 = *not at all*; 3 = *moderately*; 5 = *to a great extent*. From *Therapists' attitudes regarding the communication of positive regard* [Paper presentation], by B. A. Farber and D. Ort, 2021, Society for Psychotherapy Research Annual Meeting. Copyright 2021 by B. A. Farber and D. Ort. Reprinted with permission.

one likes a client are two of the most common forms of therapist dishonesty (Jackson et al., 2022). Thus, it may be the case that whereas many therapists do not believe they have to like their clients to convey PR, they may still believe it necessary to act as though they do.

Alternatively, therapists may feel that they can be positively regarding even if they do not actually like their clients. They may feel a general sense of respect for their clients and believe they can work effectively even with individuals they do not particularly like or would certainly not like outside of the therapeutic setting. From this perspective, the therapist's job is not to like clients but rather to work with them to achieve their goals. All seasoned therapists have almost certainly had the experience of working with clients whose past actions toward others (e.g., domestic violence, poor parenting), or even current behavior in sessions, makes liking them difficult but whose commitment to therapy makes them worthy recipients of support, acceptance, and respect.

Finally, whereas one might assume that PR—typically associated with a consistent sense of warmth, caring, acceptance, and respect—goes hand in hand with "liking," it is possible that many therapists view "liking" their clients as extending beyond the boundaries of PR, as occupying a more personal space than they feel comfortable with in a professional therapeutic relationship. As we noted previously (see Chapter 1), liking or explicitly affirming clients implies a conditionality that goes against the grain of traditional person-centered therapists and many outside this orientation, as well. Rogers himself did not typically invoke "liking" in describing what he meant by PR, preferring more neutral and somewhat less personally evaluative terms like "acceptance," "caring," and "prizing."

In addition to investigating therapists' perceptions of the overall importance of PR and their sense of which aspects of PR they and their clients especially valued, we wanted to know the extent to which therapists believed the provision of PR affects the strength of the therapeutic relationship and positive therapeutic outcome. Therapists in our sample strongly endorsed the belief that PR directly impacts the therapeutic relationship and treatment outcome, with mean scores of 4.56 ($SD = .71$) and 4.39 ($SD = .79$), respectively. The percentage of respondents endorsing *to a great extent* on these questions was 91% and 86%, respectively. In a later, open-ended part of our study, our respondents provided some examples of the way they thought about these associations. Much like Yalom (see Chapter 4), one therapist wrote about his penchant for checking in about his connection to his clients—"How is our relationship feeling to you?"—suggesting that in him doing so, his clients felt positively regarded and their relationship strengthened. Another respondent reported that asking her client, "Is there anything I can do to help you feel more supported or comfortable?" conveyed a strong sense of PR, in turn strengthening the bond between them and increasing the client's self-esteem.

The final questions in this section of our study asked therapists to consider whether they had ever sensed a rupture in the therapeutic alliance that could be attributable to clients experiencing either too much or too little PR. Mean scores for these two items were relatively low: $M = 1.87$ ($SD = .93$) and $M = 2.34$ ($SD = .99$), respectively. Furthermore, 60% of our sample endorsed low scores (either 1 or 2 on the 5-point scale) in response to the question of whether they had ever sensed an alliance rupture attributable to clients feeling too little PR. An even greater proportion—76% of our sample—endorsed one of these low rating points in response to the question of whether they had ever sensed a rupture attributable to clients experiencing too much PR.

By contrast, in an earlier, qualitative study (Suzuki, 2018), clients indicated the belief that PR could be overdone, resulting in the provision of PR feeling disingenuous or cloying. In that study, clients also described therapeutic relationships that had been hindered by a lack of PR in the form of poor attunement, inappropriate or rigid boundaries, or therapists' combative or judgmental tone. One possible explanation for this lack of convergence in therapists' and clients' views is that clients in this previous study (constituting a much smaller sample) had less skillful, well-attuned therapists than were represented in the current study—that the therapists surveyed in this most recent (Farber & Ort, 2021) study were, on the whole, more competent clinicians, more consistently able to provide effective relational elements. Another possibility is that therapists are simply not accurate raters of their own performance or of their clients' experience. That is, they may believe either that they are consistently achieving more-or-less optimal levels of PR when they are not or, somewhat more benignly, that potential deviations from these levels are short-term and eminently fixable, not dramatic enough to result in a rupture. However, in light of this discrepancy, it seems prudent for therapists to consider that the precision and degree of the PR they convey may be more impactful than realized and, when excessive or underdone, may lead to client distress or even ruptures in the therapeutic alliance.

Yet another reason therapists tend not to associate too much or too little PR with alliance ruptures may lie in the fact that they are often unaware of their patients' frustration. In fact, several participants in the smaller, qualitative study indicated that they never addressed their sense of inadequate PR directly with their therapist. As noted earlier, one of the most common issues about which patients are dishonest are their true feelings about their therapist and the therapeutic relationship (Farber, Blanchard, & Love, 2019). Therapists may simply not be aware when their attempts at PR go awry. In a similar vein, therapists may not sufficiently appreciate the extent to which individual differences, including those related to identity issues, play a role in the way different clients apprehend different aspects and degrees of PR. Therapists may consider PR as fundamentally important but still underestimate the need to tailor its specific expressions to the needs of specific clients at specific moments of treatment.

More generally, the discrepancy between client and therapist understanding of the potential of PR to be insufficiently or excessively conveyed underscores the reality that therapists' understanding of the effects of PR may not always accord with their clients' experience. Because many clients are loath to share their feelings about their therapist, their relationship, and the effectiveness of their treatment, it may well prove useful for therapists to directly inquire of their clients as to how they are experiencing their therapists' means and style of conveying PR (e.g., "I know I often check with you to see whether I fully understand what you are trying to express to me—I am wondering how this feels to you," "I'm wondering how you experienced my complimenting you on that achievement of yours"). The positive consequences of this kind of meta-communication will likely be twofold: Not only will the therapist provide a space within which clients can voice any concerns or course correct how they would like to receive PR, but checking in on how clients feel about PR might also be, in itself, a way of conveying it.

PSYCHOTHERAPISTS' PERCEPTIONS OF SPECIFIC ACTIONS AND BEHAVIORS THAT CONVEY POSITIVE REGARD

As we have discussed throughout this book, Rogers was quite consistent in his belief that PR is essentially an attitude reflective of the therapist's beliefs about being in relationship to others, rather than a set of specific behaviors. To this end, Rogers (1951) wrote, "the words—of either client or counselor—are seen as having minimal importance compared with the present emotional relationship that exists between the two" (p. 172). His contention that words and actions are only minimally important is, in our view, not exactly right, as most of the 540 clients surveyed in our lab's previous study (Suzuki & Farber, 2016) reported feeling highly affirmed by a wide range of therapist behaviors and statements.

Thus, as a follow-up to this previous (Suzuki & Farber, 2016) study, we investigated therapists' perceptions of the most affirming and most often employed aspects of PR. To do so, we adapted the Psychotherapist Expressions of Positive Regard scale (PEPR; Suzuki & Farber, 2016) and presented therapists with 29 different actions (e.g., "I smile at my clients") and 15 different statements (e.g., "Good to see you") that might convey an attitude of PR to clients. Therapists were then asked to rate "How good or affirming would this feel, or does it feel, to your clients?" (PEPR-Affirming scale [PEPR-A]) and "How characteristic or typical is this behavior in your work with clients?" (PEPR-Likely scale [PEPR-L]).

Findings from this study revealed that therapists, like clients, overwhelmingly perceive specific behaviors and statements as affirming. In addition, consistent with clients' views, there was significant thematic breadth to the items rated most highly by therapists. Table 7.3 shows the 10 items on this survey that therapists believe are most affirming to their clients.

Empathy

Therapists in this survey rated "empathy" as the most affirming form of PR; 97% of our sample indicated that empathy was *to a great extent* affirming to their clients. This overlap between empathy and PR was reflected, as well, by the many therapists who, in responding to an open-ended question about the different ways they convey PR, indicated that they listen to their clients with respect and empathy and, similarly, that their role is to mirror their clients' feelings and express their understanding. Clients, too, believe that empathy and therapist perspective taking are highly positively regarding (Suzuki, 2018).

We especially appreciate the way that McWilliams (2004), a contemporary psychodynamic practitioner, understands the mutative properties of empathy. Her sense is that a therapist's restatement of what a client has said, infused

TABLE 7.3. Therapists' Perceptions of the Most Affirming (Positively Regarding) Therapist Behaviors (*N* = 269)

Item	*M*	*SD*
"I empathize with my clients."	4.78	.49
"I summarize what my clients have said accurately."	4.55	.68
"I compliment my clients on something they feel is a strength of theirs."	4.54	.66
"I remember the name or the details of someone or something my clients spoke of long ago."	4.52	.84
"I make a connection between my clients' current experience and something they have discussed in the past."	4.48	.67
"I encourage my clients to take pride in the things they do well."	4.48	.70
"I show my clients I am listening through my body language."	4.42	.77
"I offer my clients a new way of understanding a part of themselves that they usually view as a weakness."	4.40	.73
"I maintain eye contact with my clients."	4.36	.78
"I laugh at my clients' funny comments."	4.31	.76

Note. Mean scores reflect scoring on a 5-point Likert-type scale wherein 1 = *not at all*; 3 = *moderately*; 5 = *to a great extent*.

with some emphasis on the feeling underneath the client's words, gives "shape and color" to the narrative: "The person's experience is not so much one of being 'reflected' as of being *organized* by the power of the words to give form to chaos" (McWilliams, 2004, p. 195). In addition, then, to being experienced as a form of caring and respect, therapists' empathy may lead to deeper levels of self-organization and greater self-awareness.

Summarizing and Remembering

Ranked as especially affirming by therapists, and quite consistent with Rogers's typical clinical behavior, were the items "I summarize what my clients have said accurately" and "I remember the name or the details of someone or something my clients spoke of long ago." As we noted in discussing the results of the client survey on PR in Chapter 6, both of these actions require a deep level of attentiveness that conveys a sense of value and care to the client.

In regard to summarizing accurately, a therapist in our sample, apparently invoking her inner Carl Rogers, shared the following:

> I ask if what I have said is an accurate statement of what they have said to me, and ask if what I have said feels accurate to their experience. I verbally acknowledge that my statement may not feel accurate to their feelings, and if so, to please help me understand further.

This form of PR communicates the therapist's sincere desire to fully understand clients' subjective experiences, while also repositioning clients as the experts of their own experience.

With respect to remembering details, one therapist wrote:

> I remember as much detail as possible in every session, and keep these in mind to refer back to when necessary, e.g., to affirm, to challenge, to help clients make potential links or insights for themselves, or to show them that I respect them enough to remember what they have said.

Another therapist shared, "The fact that I tend to remember details about their lives and bring them in seems to provide a sense of being liked, respected, cared for and held." Such validation can also be seen as a prizing of clients' experience—recalling in great detail the narrative that clients have disclosed communicates to them that their story is worth hearing and remembering.

Making Connections

Less consistent with traditional conceptions of PR but also regarded as highly affirming by both clients and therapists is the item, "I make connections between my clients' current experiences and something they have discussed in the past." Pointing out themes in clients' narratives is most often assumed to be the purview of psychodynamically oriented therapists, but therapists operating within the realm of cognitive behavior therapy often do much the same, referring to schemas rather than internalized relational or attachment patterns. That a diverse group of clinicians appreciates the highly affirmative quality of therapists' efforts to help clients see the connections between their past and present again highlights the multitude of ways that therapists can express respect, caring, and attentive listening.

Encouraging Self-Pride

Encouraging clients to take pride in the things they do well is another highly rated PR facet, per the judgment of therapists. Whereas Rogers believed strongly that the principles underlying client-centered therapy would lead to increased client self-worth and pride, he would not actively suggest to clients that they engage in this form of self-affirmation. That would be far too directive a stance for Rogers.

Encouraging self-pride in clients can be seen as providing a compliment—the therapist is recognizing a client's strength—but goes a step further by encouraging clients to recognize their own strengths and affirm their own competence. One therapist shared that this particular form of PR is especially helpful in her work with "clients who consistently look for reaffirmation" and that she encourages self-pride as a way to "reinforce that they know how to give themselves positive regard." The survey responses of therapists and clients indicated that both groups believe that this therapist action is slightly less affirming than therapists' explicit compliments. That is, telling a client, "You are very good at coping with hard feelings" seems to be thought of as slightly more affirming than "You should be proud of yourself for coping with hard feelings" or "It seems to me, you should take credit for that success of yours." Why? Perhaps the latter expressions are heard as containing subtle undertones of rebuke or judgment, as though the therapist is insinuating that the client *should* be more capable of recognizing his or her strengths, whereas the former contains a more reassuring and validating message. Thus, therapists may find it helpful to rely on other forms of PR with especially sensitive clients or with those inclined to feel criticized when encouraged to recognize their own strengths.

Body Language, Eye Contact, and Laughter

Three other items on therapists' list of top 10 most affirming actions include "showing I am listening through my body language," "maintaining eye contact with clients," and "laughing at clients' funny comments or jokes." These actions convey a level of attunement and respect that falls under the PR umbrella and were ranked as highly positively regarding by clients, as well. As our colleague Jesse Geller has wisely observed, when it comes to harnessing the transformative powers of offering a patient PR, psychotherapy is as much or even more a "looking cure" as it is a "talking cure" (J. D. Geller, personal communication, May 18, 2020).

As we noted in our discussion of client perceptions of PR, body language and eye contact are vivid and immediate indications of the therapist's warmth and attentiveness. In the current study, many therapists mentioned body language and consistent eye contact as ways to communicate to their clients "I hear you, I really do." Laughter, too, is inherently relational as well as complimentary, providing positive feedback in regard to the client's sense of humor. In addition to conveying affirmation, laughter is tied to a variety of positive therapeutic outcomes, including client perceptions of effectiveness and hope, and overall pleasure participating in therapy sessions (Panichelli et al., 2018). Like many other facets of PR, it may serve also to strengthen the therapeutic alliance and communicate to the client that they are truly liked.

DISCREPANCIES BETWEEN CLIENTS' AND THERAPISTS' RATINGS OF THE MOST POSITIVELY REGARDING THERAPIST BEHAVIORS

The results of our independent surveys of clients and therapists suggest great convergence in these groups' views of which therapist behaviors feel most positively regarding. The consensus between these samples is encouraging and speaks to therapists' general attunement with clients' PR needs. However, we also considered it prudent to statistically analyze potential differences. To do so, item scores on each of the two surveys were centered at the group mean. Negative mean scores represent a mean response below the group mean response, aggregated across all items.

Among the top-rated items, there appear to be two noteworthy discrepancies in therapist and client perceptions of the extent to which certain actions or behaviors convey PR. These two items are "I offer my clients a new way of understanding a part of themselves that they usually view as a weakness" and "I compliment my clients on something they feel is a strength of theirs." The former item was among the top 10 most affirming actions for both clients and therapists. The fact that an intervention of this sort is widely regarded as having an affirmative quality is itself remarkable, representing a significant deviation from the once-dominant view that UPR is incompatible with therapists' active attempts to help clients change their self-deprecating thoughts or feelings. However, the extent to which therapists and clients viewed this item as affirming varied. From clients' perspective, this intervention is the single most affirming therapist action on the list of the most affirming actions ($M = 0.09$, $SD = .92$); by contrast, therapists ranked this action as the eighth most affirming type of PR ($M = -0.05$, $SD = .73$). These group-centered means were statistically different, $t(767) = 2.14$, $p < .05$. The discrepancy here suggests that clients feel more affirmed when their therapist suggests new ways of understanding weaknesses than therapists may realize.

Complimenting clients on something they feel is a strength is another item that is ranked highly, by both clients and therapists, for its affirming qualities. One therapist in our sample provided an example of how compliments can convey PR: "I praise their achievements and personal strengths and the progress they make towards their goals." But this item represents an instance in which therapists believe they are providing PR at a level *higher* ($M = .09$, $SD = .66$) than clients report feeling it ($M = -02$, $SD = .96$). The discrepancy here, while not statistically significant ($p = .09$), is still intriguing. Why might compliments leave clients feeling less affirmed than therapists suspect? Perhaps for some clients, especially those struggling with low self-esteem, explicit compliments may feel gratuitous or undeserved. In line with this hypothesis, one therapist shared, "A client I saw frequently undercut compliments I gave her as well as compliments other group members gave her because she felt she 'did not deserve' them." Another possibility is that therapists may, at times, overcompliment, conceivably assuming "the more the merrier." However, as we've noted, some clients report feeling that too many compliments can feel disingenuous; therapists, therefore, need to appraise the intensity and volume of their compliments to match specific client needs. In this regard, multiple studies indicate that greater convergence within the dyad has a positive influence on the therapy process and/or treatment outcome. For example, Marmarosh and Kivlighan (2012) found that convergence between therapist and client perceptions of the working alliance was positively related to greater session smoothness as well as symptom reduction.

ACTIONS AND BEHAVIORS THERAPISTS PERCEIVE AS LEAST POSITIVELY REGARDING

The items that therapists consider *least* positively regarding include putting a hand on a client's shoulder ($M = 2.59$, $SD = 1.06$), hugging a client ($M = 2.76$, $SD = 1.08$), and shaking hands with a client ($M = 2.85$, $SD = 1.19$). These were the only items with mean scores below 3.0 on the 5-point scale. The relatively low mean scores for these behaviors likely reflect the apprehension among many therapists, in recent years, regarding the ethics and propriety of physical contact with clients. The findings of Schwartz-Mette and Shen-Miller (2018), replicating a 30-year-old study by Pope et al. (1987), confirm our sense that therapists have become increasingly sensitive to potential ethical violations in their interaction with clients, especially in regard to behaviors that include physical touch. For example, hugging or shaking hands with clients were both deemed significantly less ethical by therapists in the more recent Schwartz-Mette and Shen-Miller study than in Pope et al.'s earlier study.

These behaviors are just too likely to provide mixed signals, at certain times (or with certain patients) suggestive of caring but at other times suggestive of porous and unethical boundaries. As noted in Chapter 6, clients may experience therapists who act in these ways as either unresponsive to client needs or as crossing boundaries by prioritizing therapists' own needs. Whereas an opportunity to express an especial sense of closeness or support to a client may be lost as a result of adhering to a conservative approach, it seems prudent for therapists to assume this stance when the potential for misunderstanding or negative consequences is significant. We wonder, though, how many therapists make exceptions to avoiding any physical contact when, at the time of terminating a long-term treatment, a mutually experienced need for a hug seems more appropriate and less fraught. More generally, we wonder whether therapists in our survey, even under conditions of anonymity and confidentiality, were totally honest in acknowledging occasional (and presumably innocent) physical contact as a means of showing care and support.

POSITIVELY REGARDING ACTIONS THERAPISTS PERCEIVE AS OCCURRING MOST AND LEAST OFTEN IN THEIR CLINICAL WORK

Table 7.4 indicates that the behaviors clinicians believe are most affirming are also the ones that they suggest they are likely to partake in most frequently. Consistent with studies that show that therapists tend to be overly positive when evaluating their personal performance (Clemence et al., 2005; Walfish et al., 2012), the therapists in our sample may have rated themselves as partaking frequently in the behaviors that they believe to be most affirming. However, the extensive overlap here can also be seen as an indication of therapists' commitment to incorporating positively regarding behaviors into their clinical work. Except for the item "I laugh at my clients' funny comments," all items in the top 10 most affirming actions (see Table 7.3) were also represented in the top 10 most frequently occurring actions. A fair number of therapists may feel that laughing at remarks or quips may represent colluding with a client's defense or that such an action may feel insincere to either

TABLE 7.4. Therapists' Perceptions of the Most Frequently Occurring Affirming (Positively Regarding) Therapist Behaviors (*N* = 269)

Item	*M*	*SD*
"I empathize with my clients."	4.72	.52
"I make a connection between my clients' current experience and something they have discussed in the past."	4.60	.61
"I show my clients I am listening through my body language."	4.50	.70
"I encourage my clients to take pride in the things they do well."	4.49	.77
"I maintain eye contact with my clients."	4.47	.76
"I summarize what my clients have said accurately."	4.41	.71
"I smile at my clients."	4.37	.78
"I remember the name or the details of someone or something my clients spoke of long ago."	4.30	.74
"I compliment my clients on something they feel is a strength of theirs."	4.29	.89
"I offer my clients a new way of understanding a part of themselves that they usually view as a weakness."	4.27	.83

Note. Mean scores reflect scoring on a 5-point Likert-type scale wherein 1 = *not at all*; 3 = *moderately*; 5 = *to a great extent*.

themselves or their client. But more generally, the extensive list of interventions noted previously can serve as a resource for clinicians seeking to convey PR in a more expansive and personalized way.

Notably, too, the PR items that therapists reported as occurring least frequently in their practice were essentially identical to those items they saw as least positive regarding, including putting a hand on a client's shoulder (*M* = 1.65, *SD* = .96), hugging (*M* = 1.78, *SD* = .95), and shaking hands (*M* = 2.53, *SD* = 1.39). Other reported low-occurring behaviors included contacting clients after a particularly emotional session (*M* = 2.35, *SD* = 1.38), tearing up in response to a client's sad story (*M* = 2.48, *SD* = 1.22), and sharing something personal with a client (*M* = 2.63, *SD* = 1.04).

HOW DO THERAPISTS SHIFT THEIR PROVISION OF POSITIVE REGARD AS A FUNCTION OF CLIENT DIFFERENCES?

Even before the results of our surveys indicated as much, theoretical and clinical reports (see Chapters 1–3) suggested that much of the psychotherapeutic world had moved toward a way of thinking about PR in which diverse means of therapist expression of PR were accepted and appreciated by therapists and clients. Yet another important trend, arguably one that has taken on far greater prominence, is the growing awareness of the need for therapists to attend to issues of client diversity and identity. The third section of our study combined these two themes: investigating the extent to which therapists attend to individual differences in their provision of multiple forms of PR.

The first item in this section of the survey, "To what extent does your provision of positive regard shift as a function of the specific client you are working with?" was answered on a 5-point Likert-type scale. This was followed by an open-ended item requesting examples of clients to whom providing PR was challenging. Respondents were then asked whether any demographic or cultural characteristics of themselves or their clients affected the way they conveyed PR. Responses to these open-ended questions were systematically coded using a grounded theory approach, allowing us to identify a wide range of themes.

Respondents' mean score was 3.30 (*SD* = 1.09) on the question about the extent to which their PR shifts as a function of the client whom they are treating. Viewed through a different metric, these therapists were largely split in their opinion about the degree of this influence: slightly fewer than half (44%) endorsed *to a great extent*, a third (33%) selected *moderately*, and about a quarter (23%) chose *not at all*. The relatively low mean score on this item, reflecting a divergence of views among therapists, was surprising. By contrast, as reported earlier in this chapter, the mean score on the item reflecting the extent to which PR guides therapists' clinical work was 4.5 on the 5-point scale. Why, then, is there such a discrepancy in ratings between therapists' evaluation of how much PR guides their work and the extent to which they shift their provision of PR according to specific clients?

Perhaps the respondents who indicated that their provision of PR does not shift or only moderately shifts across clients thought that this question referred to the level or intensity of their care or support for different clients, rather than the means by which they provide PR. It is also possible that despite conveying PR through a variety of actions and statements, some therapists conceptualize PR within a more traditional frame and, consistent with the principle of unconditionality, as a mostly invariant attitude. Finally, it is possible that for some therapists, what shifts most in their work with different clients is not their actual *provision* of PR but rather the way they internally *feel* while providing PR. We have more to say about this theme later in this chapter.

THERAPISTS' PERCEPTIONS OF CLIENTS TO WHOM PROVIDING POSITIVE REGARD IS CHALLENGING

There were three overarching categories among the responses to the open-ended question asking therapists to describe the clients and associated factors that may make it challenging to provide PR. Among the 197 respondents who provided answers to this question, most (84%) cited clients who persistently resist or reject therapist-provided PR. Many (65%) also cited clients who present with a variety of symptoms associated with narcissistic, borderline, or antisocial personality disorders. A smaller group of respondents (13%) mentioned unmotivated clients who appear disengaged from the therapeutic process.

Clients Who Resist Positive Regard

Not surprisingly, therapists felt their efforts at providing PR were most challenged by clients who persistently resisted or rejected actions and behaviors reflecting this attitude. These clients could not accept their therapists' efforts to care for them, support them, and treat them respectfully. Therapists in our survey tended to understand clients' resistance to PR as stemming from low self-esteem and mistrust—the very issues that often led these clients to seek treatment in the first place. One therapist shared,

> A client recently discontinued therapy because she was frequently annoyed and angry with me when I attempted to support and empathize with her. My comments on how well she was handling a challenging situation were frequently met by her saying "It sounds like what I am dealing with is too much for you to handle."

Another recalled a patient for whom validation of her emotional experience, even simply repeating what she had just said verbatim, was experienced as an indictment: "Finding a way to support and validate her, when all attempts to connect were batted away was difficult." However, some of our respondents also reported that client resistance to PR served to generate fruitful discussions about therapy and the therapeutic relationship. According to the therapist we last quoted, "As a consequence of her [my client's] resistance, we discussed the difficulties of getting close, connecting, trust—and over time, things got closer between us."

Another clinician shared her particular struggle with clients who are "unresponsive when [PR] is provided," explaining that "a client who becomes defensive, angry, untrusting, sad, guilty, or any other action, even when that action may be negative, is far easier to maintain PR with than a client who is unresponsive at all." Whereas many therapists acknowledged feeling frustrated and discouraged in the face of client unresponsiveness or explicit rejection, the overwhelming majority of these therapists also maintained that such feelings did not lead to differences to their provision of PR nor their general demeanor in the room. The dialectic expressed here is that while therapists are still very much human, they are also acutely aware of their professional role and responsibility to act with their clients' best interests in mind. As one therapist stated, "Ironically, these [clients who resist or reject PR] are the very clients who likely need it the most."

Clients Who Display Narcissistic, Borderline, or Antisocial Traits

Many therapists in our study found it extremely difficult to provide PR to patients whose attitude and behavior—both within and outside of the therapeutic context—were described as "demeaning," "angry/aggressive," "very negative and critical of others," or simply "unkind." These patterns were often mentioned in tandem with referencing narcissistic, borderline, or antisocial personality disorders. One therapist recounted that after a patient

> yelled at me and questioned the way that I conducted the session . . . I cried, and it was really hard to genuinely like her after that. I felt myself on guard and it was harder to be warm with her.

Another felt significantly frustrated by "a client who was narcissistic. . . . It was hard to listen to her 'woe is me' stories while she continuously went about wrecking the relationships in her life." This therapist stated that she was aware that her client was triggering her but still found it "challenging to find something to like about her." A variation of this theme was reflected in the account of another therapist who found PR especially challenging in working with a "a client who tends to be self-focused and narcissistic . . . especially in regard to how he treats women."

In addition to struggling keenly with the ways these clients behaved, therapists reported being deeply affected by the apparent lack of empathy and remorse that accompanied these behaviors. As one therapist stated, "It is very difficult to maintain PR for individuals who have perpetrated sexual assault without remorse." Another described a client who suffered an alcohol relapse and then "drove, got into an accident, killed two innocent young people in another car . . . spoke defensively about the situation and dismissed some responsibility for it, which made it even harder to hold complete PR." Some therapists also described a subgroup of clients whose lack of empathy and concern for others manifested in their beliefs as opposed to their behaviors. These were clients who espoused misogynistic, racist, anti-Semitic, or nativist views during therapy sessions. One therapist, for example, admitted that she found it "difficult to empathize with people who express racist beliefs." It is quite possible that the social and political context in the United States at the time this survey was deployed (e.g., the 2020 election and the murder of George Floyd) exacerbated the extent to which therapists experienced these beliefs as offensive.

The overall challenges of providing PR to clients within this group differed from those mentioned in the previous "resistant" category. Whereas therapists dealing with resistance were frustrated because their attempts at providing PR were persistently rejected, therapists here struggled to provide PR while feeling dismayed with the overall way these clients related to others. Clients whose behaviors do not elicit authentic acceptance, respect, and empathy highlight the challenge posed by the "unconditional" component of Rogerian PR.

At first blush, therapists' difficulty in providing PR to clients with personality disorders and/or racist or misogynistic views suggests what may be an implicit prerequisite for the conveyance of this attitude—that the client is at least minimally caring about others. However, as is the case with resistant clients, therapists in our survey generally insisted that they strove to minimize judgmental feelings, even with truly difficult clients. One way that therapists facilitated PR under these circumstances was to focus on exploring the origins of clients' problematic behaviors. One therapist, presumably someone with a psychodynamic bent, noted that she was able to find a way to provide PR to a "misogynistic and condescending" client by exploring the root of these behaviors and reaching his more vulnerable core.

Therapists' commitment to find *something* to like in every client was also cited as a way to abate frustration and effectively provide PR. One therapist suggested that his work with "rude, unkind, or stubborn" clients did not interfere with his PR because he "always finds something to like or respect about them, even if it's how creatively they insulted me." Another therapist shared that in her work with challenging and confrontational clients, she pictures them as a young child in order to feel empathy and compassion. Yet another therapist reported that he simply reminds himself that "clients who are angry or abusive can be challenging but that is when compassion is most effective."

Some of our respondents also mentioned specific modifications to their provision of PR in working with difficult clients. For example, with a client who reported that women are often emotionally injured by his behaviors, one therapist reported "caringly challenging" him to consider other ways of interacting. Another therapist invoked a similar modification with clients presenting with features of narcissistic personality disorder:

> In that situation, it is necessary to employ empathic confrontation to help the patient understand how their behavior affects others. As rapport develops, it becomes possible to join and provide positive regard to the more vulnerable, hidden parts of the patient's self.

Clients Who Are Unmotivated

Many therapists also struggle to provide PR to clients described as "unmotivated." These are individuals who appear disengaged from the therapeutic process and uninterested in deepening the relationship. They may be unmotivated as a result of being in therapy by court order, parental force, or ulterior motives such as obtaining medication or financial assistance. One therapist recounted the case of a client who was in treatment only because his mother insisted upon it. "She wants him there so he's not receptive to much of what we do in session, so it's tough to praise him and empathize with him when he's not giving me much to work with." Another therapist wrote of his particular frustration with clients who seemed "stuck" on taking action to change their situation: "It didn't much change my positive regard of them but did make me think about taking different approaches and wonder whether my positive regard was in some way enabling the 'stagnancy.'"

Whereas these clients differ from those in the resistant category—they are not actively antagonistic to PR—they seem to elicit a similar dilemma for therapists. How best to provide PR to clients who seem to struggle to accept it or profit from it? Although most therapists in our survey suggested that they were almost invariably able to be positively regarding to resistant, difficult, and/or disengaged clients, it seems likely that the client's engagement in the treatment process must influence, at least somewhat, the extent to which therapists can genuinely convey this attitude. Carl Rogers was exceptional in his ability to convey PR to even the most difficult, intransigent, seductive, and nonreactive clients (Farber et al., 1996; see especially the case of "A Silent Young Man"). But not every therapist is Carl Rogers.

CLIENT IDENTITY AND THERAPIST PROVISION OF POSITIVE REGARD

In addition to investigating which client characteristics make it challenging for therapists to provide PR, we also inquired as to whether, and in what ways, clients' identity-related characteristics (e.g., race, age, gender, ethnicity, sexual orientation) affect the provision of PR. An analysis of the responses provided by the 163 respondents who answered this question revealed that the majority (60%) modify the ways they provide PR to clients who differ in some salient way from themselves. Some in this group also took pains to distinguish between levels of PR and the means to convey this attitude:

> I try to exhibit the same level of positive regard for patients regardless of any particular characteristics, while also trying to be mindful of any biases I have that may affect my interactions with clients, and may change my style based on a client's needs.

A smaller group of respondents to this question (22%) reported that clients' demographic and cultural factors were irrelevant to their provision of PR.

It is not surprising that the majority of therapists in our sample acknowledged clients' demographic and cultural factors as affecting their provision of PR. In recent decades, the importance of multicultural awareness and competency has garnered extensive recognition across a range of disciplines, including psychotherapy. Also not surprising, and very consistent with the contemporary zeitgeist, is that these respondents emphasized identity-related differences within the therapist–patient dyad rather than specific client variables.

These therapists' sense was that salient differences between themselves and their client—for example, around age, gender, ethnicity, or sexual orientation—needed to be taken into consideration in deciding how to convey PR. Several respondents suggested that therapists should, early in therapy, monitor how their communicative style is working for the client—a process that many noted should always happen but one that is particularly important in instances where there are salient individual differences between the therapist and client. Other therapists in our study acknowledged engaging in more overt displays of PR in certain circumstances: "When there are obvious [demographic and cultural] differences between me and my client, I am generally more intentional and aware of expressing positive regard in demonstrable and noticeable ways." However, therapists cautioned against excessive, overt displays of PR, with one therapist stating,

> It is easy for me to be intimidated by clients whose race, gender, or ethnicity are not congruent with mine, which may lead to an overcorrection (almost frantically so) of positive regard. This can feel disingenuous for clients, I think.

Too much PR, even well intentioned, runs the risk of being perceived as insincere or even condescending by clients. The PR in question here is not of that basic acceptance variety but rather of those more explicitly affirming and complimentary forms.

Gender (i.e., mixed-gender dyad) emerged as the most frequently cited client–therapist difference (32%) affecting therapists' provision of PR. Although some therapist responses referred to gender exclusively (e.g., "I am way less likely to tell male clients that I am proud of them"), gender was most often discussed in tandem with sexual orientation and within the context of avoiding flirtatious or mixed messages. For example, one therapist explained that he was "careful to make sure that positive regard does not come across as flirting with patients whose sexual orientation means they prefer my gender."

Race and ethnicity were also frequently noted (28%) as differences that may impact PR. Therapists in our sample were far from unanimous in considering how best to modify their PR in cases of cross-racial dyads. Some, as noted previously, suggested that they were likely to provide more overt displays of PR; others argued strongly that this position was intrinsically demeaning, even racist; and still others held to the belief that "one size never fits all" and that the provision of PR, like the provision of all clinical interventions and attitudes, must depend on the specific dynamics of a given therapist–client dyad.

Age discrepancy was cited by 20% of respondents as a factor affecting therapist PR. Some therapists noted, for example, that in comparison with working with an older client, they would likely approach a younger client with more warmth and praise, modify their language to include more humor, and even "throw a curse word in there to help them feel more comfortable." On the other hand, in their work with older clients, some suggested that they were more apt to provide PR by highlighting the client's life experiences, "trying to be more sweet," and, specifically, "not cursing." With regard to age differences in which the therapist is significantly older than the client, clinicians often shared the sense that their PR was especially likely to be perceived as "warm" and "maternal."

Some therapists advocated for identity-related differences to be addressed as part of the therapeutic process and suggested that the therapist's responsibility is to initiate such dialogues. Many recommended acknowledging differences up-front and discussing them openly with new clients. One therapist shared the following:

> I approach these factors with a sense of curiosity; as if I am the student and the individual is the professor who gets to teach me about a subject they know very well: their unique self. If anything, these factors often improve the way I provide positive regard, as it allows me to effectively demonstrate my acceptance and genuine interest in the person.

Although in some ways this feels true to the Rogerian client-as-expert credo, Rogers himself would likely not have actively pursued his curiosity in this direct a manner. In perhaps the best example of him working in individual therapy with a racially different (African American) client (Whiteley, 1977), Rogers is accepting and empathic, frequently checking his understanding of his client's narrative. But he does not comment on their racial difference or explore how this difference affects their relationship. His steadfast belief, manifest in this demonstration session, is to assume, as much as possible, another's perspective:

> We fail to see that we are evaluating the person from our own, or from some fairly general, frame of reference, but that the only way to understand his behavior meaningfully is to understand it as he perceives it himself, just as the only way to understand another culture is to assume the frame of reference of that culture. (Rogers, 1951, p. 494)

As most therapists strove to adjust PR to address identity-related differences between themselves and their clients, many also indicated that dyadic similarities had an effect on PR, as well. Per the words of one of our respondents: "I may unintentionally relate better with those who have more similar characteristics to myself and thus may find it easier to provide understanding, PR, etc." Another therapist explained that shared gender and sexual minority status help facilitate PR, as "it is sometimes easier for me to connect with patients who are also sexual/gender minorities like me. PR might come a little bit more naturally with these clients as we are members of the same 'community.'" Some therapists also found that PR was easier to impart to clients with similar cultural backgrounds. As one noted, "It's easier to use helpful cultural phrases and words with patients from my own cultural background." Importantly, though, she added, "But this affects only the way in which I provide positive regard, not the amount or extent of positive regard that I provide."

Finally, it is important to note that some, albeit a minority, of the therapists in our survey asserted that demographic and cultural factors did not affect their provision of PR. Somewhat provocatively, one therapist indicated that "multicultural factors are irrelevant as far as PR is concerned." Those who held to this position contended that adjusting one's therapeutic style due to demographic or cultural factors violated their ethical framework. For example, one therapist shared her sense that "as therapists, we need to be 'all in' with clients regardless of these multicultural factors. . . . Human being to human being." These therapists consistently reflected the notion that modifications to PR based on demographic or cultural factors were inherently inequitable.

Taken together, our qualitative explorations suggest that most therapists are exceedingly considerate of multicultural issues in their provision of PR. Specifically, cultural sensitivity was demonstrated in therapists' awareness of clients' demographic and cultural identity, their acknowledgment that differences within the dyad may influence clients' experience of PR, and their attempts to implement culturally responsive modifications to their provision of PR. These findings correspond to the core multicultural competencies identified in Sue et al.'s (2019) influential text. Fewer therapists stated that multicultural factors had no effect on their provision of PR—a view presumably rooted in a desire to see oneself as nondiscriminatory or even an ally but one no longer seen as culturally sensitive.

It should also be noted that our sample of therapists was primarily White, female, heterosexual, and from the United States. Lacking diversity in this sample, we were unable to adequately study how therapists of color, male therapists, those identifying as sexual minorities, or those from other countries view and tailor their communication of PR to clients who self-identify in similarly salient (or divergent) ways. As the need for cultural sensitivity increasingly takes root in clinical practice, the need for clinical and empirical reports on ways in which diversity influences the practice and receipt of

PR becomes ever more pressing. One exception to the general paucity of literature in this area was a clinical investigation of the use of person-centered therapy with impoverished, maltreated, and neglected children in Brazil (Freire et al., 2005). According to the authors, this was a quite successful trial, one in which therapists were responsive to the differing needs of the individual children, and one that confirmed Rogers's (1959) fundamental notion that "it is the therapist's unconditional acceptance of the client's experiential world that ultimately promotes growth and therapeutic change" (p. 234).

CONCLUSION

The findings presented in this chapter indicate that an eclectic group of therapists considers PR to be a central component of the therapy process and treatment outcome. In addition, this research shows that, for the most part, therapists and clients are in accord regarding which specific therapist behaviors and statements are most and least affirming. Finally, these analyses provide a preliminary understanding of how individual, identity-related differences among clients may influence therapists' provision of PR. Taken together, these findings emphasize the importance for clinicians to appreciate PR as a dynamic process, continually considering the optimal types and levels of this attitude that are best suited for a particular client at a particular time.

More specifically, the research conducted on client and therapist perceptions of PR leads to several "best practice" recommendations for clinicians of all orientations. Therapists, we believe, should strive to incorporate the most affirming forms of PR into their work, tailoring them, of course, to the needs of individual clients at given moments of therapy. These means of effectively conveying PR include empathizing with the client, accurately summarizing what the client has said, complimenting strengths, remembering names and details important to the client, making connections between current and past experiences, reframing qualities the client may perceive as weaknesses, and encouraging pride in things the client does well. Beyond these mostly verbal interventions, clinicians should also bear in mind that body language and eye contact are other meaningful ways to convey acceptance, support, and warmth. The research also suggests that therapists should be encouraged to challenge clients' existing narratives as a means of conveying PR. Although this practice seems antithetical to Rogerian tenets regarding the importance of unconditional acceptance, for a great many clients, it seemingly has the feel of "My therapist cares enough to help me change the inaccurate or invalid views I've had of myself." In fact, clients consider their therapists' "offer[ing] a new way of understanding a part of themselves that they usually view as a weakness" as the most affirming clinical intervention.

It is more difficult to offer recommendations regarding such behaviors as putting a hand on the client's shoulder, hugging, shaking hands, and sharing something personal with the client. While these behaviors—in certain circumstances—may leave some clients feeling affirmed, the potential for these behaviors to be regarded as inappropriate seems significant and fraught with the possibility of unforeseen and unfortunate consequences. With these practices in particular, therapists should be acutely aware of the need to communicate PR in accord with their clients' needs and with the best interests of their clients in mind.

In order to obtain a deeper, more contextualized sense of the way PR plays out in the therapy room, in Chapter 8 we provide examples of how PR was communicated to four different therapy clients over the course of distinct treatment modalities.

8 CLINICAL EXAMPLES OF POSITIVE REGARD IN FOUR DIFFERENT THERAPIES

Ring the bells that still can ring/Forget your perfect offering
There is a crack, a crack in everything/That's how the light gets in

—Leonard Cohen, "Anthem"

One dilemma in attempting to delineate the specifics of positive regard (PR) is the fact that, at its heart, PR is really about a pervasive attitude rather than a discrete behavior or even an affirming phrase on the part of the therapist. That is, while a therapist—or parent, spouse, or friend—can certainly find the right words that, in the moment, sound and even feel affirming, accepting, and/or supportive, if that person fails to consistently maintain that attitude, those initial words will have minimal lasting impact. In fact, over time, the person whose tendency is to be critical rather than affirming is likely to lose credibility; their attempts at momentary PR may well feel disingenuous and be met with caution or suspicion. Stated otherwise, it is hard to feel truly valued by someone who is accepting and supportive only sporadically and/or when they find it opportune. Intermittent reinforcement may keep a rat pushing a lever for food or keep a gambler at a slot machine, but intermittent

https://doi.org/10.1037/0000312-009
Understanding and Enhancing Positive Regard in Psychotherapy: Carl Rogers and Beyond,
by B. A. Farber, J. Y. Suzuki, and D. Ort

affirmation and acceptance when interspersed with indifference or criticism is not fertile soil for the growth or healing of the human spirit or a person's belief in their worth.

The major point here is that providing examples of words or behaviors that typically convey a sense of PR may be useful but fails to characterize fully the essence of Rogers's meaning: that to make a difference, the therapist's PR must be consistent, nearly invariant. It must be so to counteract the effects of experiencing chronic conditions of worth—of feeling valued contingently, superficially, and/or inconsistently. Thus, presenting a list of positively regarding actions, highlighting excerpts from individual sessions, or even reviewing transcripts of entire sessions may provide useful glimpses of the crux of this attitude but cannot convey the client's experience of enduring and consistent acceptance, nonjudgment, warmth, and support. What clients perceive as the most potent forms of PR need to be consistently imparted by therapists over the course of treatment. Discrete statements and therapist behaviors, we're suggesting, will serve as PR in a Rogerian fashion only if the attitude underlying specific instances of caring and support is abiding.

Therapists, we assume, often have a preferred way or style of providing PR, but they can also effectively mix and match specific forms of PR—a strong emphasis on empathy one session, demonstrating great interest and caring by pulling together disparate strands of a client's narrative into a coherent thread in another session, explicit statements of support in another—as long as an overall attitude of PR is maintained. Furthermore, these PR combinations are likely to change both as a function of the type of client a therapist is working with and the focus and tone of individual therapy sessions. As Stiles et al. (1998) maintained, effective therapists of all types are responsive to the changing dynamics of clients within sessions and over the course of therapy.

To provide some sense of how the various iterations of PR get expressed over the course of psychotherapy, we've included several examples. The first is from Rogers himself, working with a 20-year-old depressed client (Mary Jane Tilden) over the course of 11 sessions (Farber et al., 1996; Snyder, 1947). The second example is based on the long-term eclectic treatment, conducted by the senior author (BAF), of a woman dealing with the consequences of early parental abuse (Farber & Suzuki, 2018). The third example is based on a client's book-length account of her own long-term, primarily psychodynamic therapy dealing with issues of grief, suicidality, and abuse (Wise, 2012). The fourth and final example is a treatment in which PR is provided by a cognitive behavior therapy (CBT) practitioner (Wenzel, 2016), offered to counterbalance the reality that virtually all available examples of PR are based on the perspectives of therapists or clients in either person-centered, contemporary psychodynamic, or integrative treatments.

Although these examples are infused with consistent doses of the therapist's PR, the specific nature of the PR that each therapist offers differs significantly. Moreover, it is impossible to determine the extent to which PR, either by itself or in combination with other variables (e.g., the overall strength of the therapeutic relationship, specific psychodynamic or CBT-oriented interventions), contributed to the effectiveness of these treatments.

POSITIVE REGARD AND CLIENT-CENTERED THERAPY: THE CASE OF MARY JANE TILDEN

Mary Jane Tilden, a White female client aged 20, who had graduated high school and briefly held a job before leaving the workforce, was in therapy with Rogers from October 1946 to February 1947. She came to her first few appointments accompanied by her mother, who had called in advance expressing concerns about her daughter's depressive, withdrawn behavior. Rogers's work over the 11 sessions with Mary Jane, as she is referred to in his summary of their treatment (Farber et al., 1996; Snyder, 1947), is in many ways a classic example of his early client-centered approach. Rogers's write-up of the case consists of some segments of verbatim transcript and some narrative summary with clinical impressions. Having access to the words of Rogers and his client over the entirety of this brief course of treatment allows us to see how PR played out in his work and to surmise how it may have contributed to Mary Jane's progress in therapy.

In their first interview, Mary Jane offered a vivid sense of how lost she felt. Her very first utterance in therapy: "I can't find myself. Everything I do seems to be wrong. I can't get on with people. If there is any criticism or anyone says anything about me I just can't take it" (Farber et al., 1996, p. 144). She went on to describe a perpetual experience of "self-condemnation," whereby she compared herself with others and always felt inferior. She expressed her sense that she could not socialize and feel "natural," believing that she was behind her peers romantically and professionally, was not particularly smart or capable, and that it seemed futile to go on living.

The approach taken by Rogers seemed to have enabled Mary Jane to get to the heart of her hopeless feelings quickly. From the start, he declined to define Mary Jane's presenting problems, even though her mother had called ahead and described the issues she believed her daughter was struggling with and even though her mother reiterated these and other concerns in greater detail when accompanying Mary Jane to the first appointment. As though none of this preamble had occurred, Rogers opened the interview with the statement "I really know very little as to why you came in. Would you like to tell me something about it?" (Farber et al., 1996, p. 144). Although his client presented with all the markers of a major depressive episode, Rogers made no attempt in this or any of their sessions to label her affliction or provide her with a possible diagnosis, instead focusing on understanding her experience and amplifying her feelings about her condition (J. D. Geller & Gould, 1996). His emphasis on his client's autonomy and subjectivity came to the fore toward the end of the first session, when he engaged her in an "informed consent" conversation about counseling:

> I think it's up to you whether or not you think it's worth trying—and all that I can say is that a number of people have tried that sort of thing and have found that it helped, but you can't be guaranteed anything. It might help or it might not. I think you're wondering whether anything might help. (Farber et al., 1996, p. 151)

After grappling with this question and elaborating on her hopeless outlook, which Rogers continued to empathically reflect back to her, Mary Jane concluded that she would return the following week.

In Sessions 2 and 3, Mary Jane continued to express her ambivalence about the therapeutic process, with Rogers continuing to respond to her doubts with his signature blend of warmth and unconditional acceptance. A relational psychodynamic practitioner might highlight Mary Jane's attempts to draw Rogers into an enactment—the unconscious playing out of old patterns—as she made repeated bids for reassurance and guidance. Rogers handled these attempts in a consistently nondirective fashion. In the second interview, when Mary Jane queried, "Do you really think you could help me in any way? I mean, do you feel as though you can?" Rogers replied,

> I think I would have to leave it that—a—it comes back to the question—do you feel you want to work on it? If you do, we'll save time next week. If you feel that it is so hopeless that nothing can be done . . . (p. 156)

Rogers never completed this sentence, but as his words trailed off, Mary Jane seemed to consider his response quite seriously, pausing before she decided she would like to return: "It's really all in my own attitude, isn't it? *(Pause)* O.K. Let's make it next week, then" (Farber et al., 1996, p. 156–157). Similarly, at a key moment of exploration in the third interview, Mary Jane demanded, "Well, what's the answer? Am I supposed to get the answers?" and Rogers responded, "You're wondering that, too, aren't you, whether maybe the answer is in you?" (p. 158).

Mary Jane, so accustomed to leaning on the guidance and standards of others, did not express dismay at her therapist's apparent unwillingness to provide answers. Rather, his reply opened space for her to continue to muse about what it would take, and what it would mean, for her to make a change in her life while being unsure of the outcome. One gets the sense that these responses by Rogers, which easily could be perceived by a cynic as a rhetorical dodge or a tactic to secure the client's investment in therapy, rather flowed from a genuine conviction that Mary Jane's prognosis depended entirely on her ability to tap into her self-actualizing tendency. At the foundation of these communications were her therapist's deep respect and faith in his client's own agency and capacity for self-healing.

Rogers demonstrated this kind of regard for Mary Jane's autonomy not only in the content of his interventions within their interviews but also in his respect for the frame and integrity of the therapy as evidenced in the intersession communication that occurred between the third and fourth interviews. Mary Jane's mother contacted Rogers to inform him that her daughter was hesitating about attending their fourth visit and that she (the mother) was unsure about the adequacy of this treatment and would like a referral to a psychiatrist. Rogers demurred on this point and decided to write a note to Mary Jane voicing acceptance and understanding about her hesitation, informing her that he would hold an appointment slot for her for a few days. Mary Jane telephoned Rogers by the date he had put aside, confirming that she would keep this appointment. One imagines that it was both Rogers's acceptance of and openness to any outcome that ultimately contributed to Mary Jane's decision to return to treatment. The remarkable piece here is the ability of Rogers, likely stemming from his supportive attitude and consistent conveyance of empathy, to transform words that could well have been experienced as a noncommittal "whatever" response into a communication that felt respectful and caring. From this point onwards, though Mary Jane would continue to express some doubts about her progress, she seemed increasingly committed to the process of therapy.

As Mary Jane continued treatment, she expressed an excruciating degree of self-loathing and despair. Rogers's handling of this content is notable. He never downplayed her experience, never asked her to offer evidence for the validity of her thoughts, and never offered a reassuring reframing of her feelings. His response was essentially one of empathy and acceptance:

MARY JANE: I even feel I ought to be in a sanitarium. There must be something awfully wrong with me.

C.R.: Things have been so bad you feel perhaps you're really abnormal. (Farber et al., 1996, p. 144)

At a key moment in Session 9, Rogers and Mary Jane worked together using the power of metaphor to allow Mary Jane to access more deeply her sadness about how inhibited and unsure she had felt all her life:

C.R.:   You feel very deeply about it, that even a little child feels so much pleasure in standing on his own two feet.

MARY JANE: Well, possibly being—oh, dear, here comes the rainstorm. *(Cries)*

C.R.:   They say the rain makes things grow. (Farber et al., 1996, p. 183)

With this exchange, which Mary Jane followed with an extended period of weeping, she was able to open the door to her grief, with her therapist's PR having allowed her to pace the experience in a way that suited her best. Lest we imagine that Rogers's nondirective approach was designed with the sole goal of accessing painful emotions, we must also highlight that he just as notably followed his client's lead in the very next session, when she wished to titrate her sadness:

C.R.:   The old doubt that you could be worthwhile to anyone else. You still feel that your friendship doesn't offer very much to anyone else.

MARY JANE: *(Crying)* Here we go again. That always gets me.

C.R.:   And the tears come because you don't feel as though you really are good for anything to anyone else.

MARY JANE: That's right. It's so silly.

C.R.:   You think it's foolish to weep a little.

MARY JANE: That's right. Let's talk about something else.

C.R.:   All right. (Farber et al., 1996, p. 187)

A psychodynamic therapist with a classic bent, perhaps accustomed to seeing such a client communication as an expression of resistance, might claim that Rogers's acceptance here had the effect of colluding with the client's defenses. Practitioners of a wide range of orientations, in fact, are steeped in the idea that the true goal of therapy is to "go for the affect at all costs" and may have balked at the idea of leaving this material on the table rather than exploring further. Rogers chose to respect his client's wishes and feelings.

Rogers had a laser-like focus on illuminating the beliefs, feelings, and experiences Mary Jane brought to their sessions, most of which, especially in the first half of the treatment, were recent or present-moment focused. He made little attempt to synthesize or explore the details of her life history or even to understand the context informing her statements and assessments, instead holding to his belief that she was the master of the meaning of her own experience. When Mary Jane did reference her earlier history, including some experiences she recalled from her school days and her time working, Rogers accepted them and made no attempt to dig deeper.

This stance may feel particularly foreign to a psychodynamic sensibility, which would have Rogers explore the origins of Mary Jane's patterns and work toward an understanding of the conflicts that arose from these experiences. Indeed, J. D. Geller and Gould's (1996) commentary on this case argued that "this self-imposed restriction had an inhibitory influence on the immediacy and depth of Mary Jane's functioning during her therapy sessions" (p. 222). One might counter, though, that ultimately the client found her way to this process on her own, accessing emotional experience on her own terms. She began to reflect on the challenges of her relationship with her mother in Session 7 and her father in Session 8 and continued to deepen her insight into the origins of her difficulties and her relationship to her family in later sessions. These developments seemed to unfold in tandem with increased initiative in her social and professional life, steps that she reported to Rogers after she had taken them, without his taking on any explicit role in their planning or execution, as perhaps a cognitive behavior therapist might have done earlier in treatment.

Whereas for the most part Rogers studiously retained his stance of unconditional acceptance, thereby freeing Mary Jane to map out her own actions and make her own assessments, perhaps just as significant was his occasional departure from this stance. At the conclusion of their first session, when Mary Jane was struggling with the question of whether she wished to return for a second interview, Rogers offered some indirect reassurance that she could be helped:

MARY JANE: I don't know whether this would help me any. I mean I don't know whether anything would help me. (*Pause*) Have you ever had cases that were this bad? (*Laughs*) Or anywhere near this bad?

C.R.:   You're coming back to that question again, aren't you—wondering—well, I could answer that question—yes. (Farber et al., 1996, p. 154)

In their final session, too, Rogers was more directly supportive, even complimentary. In this session, Mary Jane was assessing her progress:

MARY JANE: So you see I've come a long way. I've faced some of these things. I've realized I'm not so bright, but I have begun to think I can get along anyway.

C.R.: Yes, you have come a long way and you really have faced some of these things pretty deeply. (Farber et al., 1996, p. 192)

This phrasing introduced Rogers's own attitude of approval and appreciation toward his client. It does not appear, from the transcript, that Mary Jane noticed this shift, as she continued with the session much as before. One might reasonably wonder why Rogers chose this moment to express these sentiments. It is not until much later in the session that Mary Jane concluded that she would like to "leave it this way" (Farber et al., 1996, p. 197), holding open the option of whether she would schedule another appointment in the future as needed (ultimately only returning about a year after this session, following some personal setbacks and a relapse into her old thought patterns). Whether Rogers had sensed this impending closure, early in the session, is unclear, but his final statement to her more or less recapitulated this expression of frankly positive appraisal: "You really have come a long way in your thinking, haven't you?" (Farber et al., 1996, p. 197).

We can imagine that Rogers had grown quite fond of his young client in their time working together. It seems that as much as he supported and respected Mary Jane's autonomy, he also had come to take pride in her growth and to feel real affection for her. The genuineness of his warmth likely infused their treatment in ways not easily captured by a transcript, save for this small utterance in their last session of this treatment course. Rogers may have refrained more than once from making more explicitly supportive and reassuring interventions, believing that his restraint was critical for her own self-actualizing tendency to revive and flourish. Nonetheless, the nonverbal expressions of warmth that doubtless emerged in the course of their brief time together may have been just as critical as his acceptance, support, and empathy, all of which seemed to allow Mary Jane to emerge from treatment with a nascent sense of vitality and confidence.

POSITIVE REGARD AND INTEGRATIVE PSYCHOTHERAPY: THE CASE OF CAROLE

In a book chapter ("Affirming the Case for Positive Regard") written by two of this book's coauthors, Farber and Suzuki (2018) provided an account of the senior author's work with a long-term psychotherapy client. That chapter focused specifically on the multiple ways in which Farber, self-identified as an integrative therapist blending aspects of client-centered and relational psychodynamic therapy, conveyed his PR for his client, "Carole," over the course of a treatment that lasted nearly a decade. Here, we provide a summary of that work.

Carole, a 25-year-old, recently divorced White woman from a working-class Irish family, presented to therapy with complaints of chronic anxiety, suicidal ideation, sleep difficulties, and uncertainty associated with her career goals. She also reported several instances of becoming blackout drunk, which occasionally led to one-night stands with strangers. Although the distress of her recent divorce prompted Carole to seek therapy, it was the pain she endured during her childhood and adolescence that became the focus of treatment. Carole recounted horrifying details of physical and sexual abuse inflicted by her father and abetted by her mother, who was either unable or unwilling to protect her. For the first few months of treatment, Carole relayed the awful details of her abuse, trying to alleviate the feelings of guilt and shame that followed her into adulthood. "She wore the scars of these acts as so many do," Farber noted, "barely ever feeling good enough or that someone could value her" (Farber & Suzuki, 2018, p. 216).

Carole's struggles to feel good about herself emerged throughout treatment. In one instance, she criticized herself for taking care of her elderly mother, claiming that her willingness to care for her mother was "a pathetic response to giving her what she doesn't deserve" (Farber & Suzuki, 2018, p. 219). In response, Farber stated that he viewed her willingness to care for her mother as a strength, not a weakness:

> I respect greatly your finding a compromise between the part of you that doesn't want to care for her at all and your sense that you don't want to act in ways that reflect either her values or those of your father. You've tried hard to be decent, to live up to your own moral values, and though it may irk you to give to her, I suspect there's a piece of you that gives yourself some credit. (Farber & Suzuki, 2018, p. 219)

Here, Farber not only affirmed Carole's worth and value as a person but went a step further by offering her an alternative and far more compassionate way of understanding a part of herself that she originally perceived as weak.

In addition to helping Carole reframe aspects of herself that she viewed as weaknesses, Farber demonstrated PR by complimenting Carole on those characteristics that she recognized as strengths. Some examples from over the years they worked together: "You've been the strength of your extended family, you've essentially held it together," "You're remarkably resilient," "That's a very smart way of looking at things," and "That's very kind of you" (Farber & Suzuki, 2018, pp. 222–223). Carole was profoundly touched by the extent to which Farber recognized her uniqueness and appreciated her strengths, and she often reacted to her therapist's words with smiles, gratitude, and even tears.

In part, Farber's explicitly affirming comments were meaningful to Carole because they touched on aspects of herself that were central to her identity.

For example, well aware of how important being a good mother was to Carole, Farber made sure to express his genuine feeling that he viewed her as a "very sensitive, loving mother" (Farber & Suzuki, 2018, p. 223). Similarly, when Carole brought some pieces of her handiwork into one of their sessions, he remarked, "You have great artistic talent" (p. 222). Overall, this type of PR, in the form of specific and timely compliments, helped Carole believe— perhaps for the first time in her life—that others recognized and valued her strengths. Note the contrast between the explicit form of PR offered here and the nonjudgmental acceptance provided by Rogers in his work with Mary Jane Tilden.

Farber often followed these positively regarding statements with a plea to Carole to credit herself for her abilities. In this way, he not only affirmed his recognition of Carole's strengths but also encouraged her to be self-affirming— a movement toward what the person-centered approach community deems unconditional positive self-regard (e.g., Murphy et al., 2020). For example, when Carole shared the details of a sensitively worded conversation she had with one of her children, Farber responded, "It's easy for me to see that you're a loving parent with really good instincts, but the task is for you to realize this" (Farber & Suzuki, 2018, p. 223). Over time, Carole did begin to internalize her strengths, eventually believing, at least to a far greater extent than previously, that she had many talents and laudable attributes. Thus, Carole's self-image improved, and despite a long history of invalidation and criticism from significant others, she began to believe more in her innate goodness.

Carole's early traumatic experiences also had an impact on her ability to trust others. Growing up, her parents regularly distorted and maligned her words and actions, leaving her with lasting fears of being hurt, disappointed, or misunderstood. How, then, did her therapist attempt to transcend these defenses and develop a secure relationship with Carole? One way was by providing Carole with accurate summaries of what she shared with him in therapy. These summaries tended to take two forms: The first, consistent with Rogers's ideas about empathic reflections, consisted of summaries of discrete statements—for example, "Winning that high school achievement award was a real turning point in your life" (Farber & Suzuki, 2018, p. 221). The second type of summary reflected the salient themes that emerged throughout their sessions. For example, after Carole repeatedly shared details of her abuse and neglect, Farber summarized, "Sounds like no one in your household really listened to you at all or believed in your worth as a human being" (p. 221). This latter sort of summarizing had an especially powerful effect on Carole, as she sensed the extent to which her therapist was attentive and fully invested in helping her make sense of her world. Overall, both types of empathic summaries enabled Carole to believe that her therapist valued her deeply enough to listen intently to what she was saying, a stark contrast from the way she was raised.

Another way Farber ensured that Carole felt heard and valued was by remembering the names of most of the important figures in Carole's life, including her immediate family members, children, and past and present significant others. Perhaps even more validating, though, was his reaction when he did forget names or details of past conversations: When Carole invoked an unfamiliar name, for example, Farber was transparent and asked Carole to remind him whom she was referring to and how this individual was important in her life. This provides a good example of how PR and genuineness—like PR and empathy—are often conflated.

Although Carole's therapist genuinely cared for her and strove to be sensitive to her needs, he inevitably erred—sometimes speaking too much, missing the point, minimizing a concern, interjecting humor to ward off his own anxieties, or questioning or interpreting when he should have been "just" listening. Apologies for these misattunements—"I'm sorry, apparently I missed the point there, didn't I?"—didn't undo them, but the apologies did seem to serve, to some extent, as another means to convey PR: They implied, "I respect you and our relationship greatly, and I'll try my best to get our work back on track."

For the most part, as treatment progressed, her therapist's consistent provision of PR helped Carole feel safer and more secure. However, not surprisingly, there were times when Carole's earlier fears of being hurt or disappointed resurfaced. When they did, Farber typically responded with some variation on phrases such as

> I understand why you'd feel like I could disappoint you—other important people in your life have certainly done so—but I'm glad we're talking about this now, I'm glad you can hear this, and I hope we can keep working on this. (Farber & Suzuki, 2018, p. 220)

These kinds of responses seemed to normalize Carole's fears and provide the space for those fears to be explored. In addition, such responses helped Carole understand the way her current fears related to her past experiences, a fundamental psychodynamic intervention but one that clients often consider within the domain of a therapist's positively regarding stance (see Chapter 6, this volume). Carole's heartfelt reply, often in the form of "Thanks for believing in me. I know I can be difficult" (Farber & Suzuki, 2018, p. 220), suggests that this type of PR—helping a client make a connection between past and present—left Carole with the belief that she was capable of working through these fears.

Consistent, too, with empirical and clinical reports that nonverbal expressions of PR are an essential aspect of this overall attitude, Carole's therapist seemed to convey PR through his posture, facial expressions, and tone of voice. Farber's sense was that he was nearly always "fully present . . . feet flat on the floor, leaning toward her, and often nodding my head to signal my understanding" (Farber & Suzuki, 2018, p. 219). In one instance, Carole shared an awful detail of her abuse, and Farber grimaced and shook his head. Carole noticed this reaction and shared with him that she perceived his facial expressions as an indication that he understood her pain. Although Rogers did not explicitly address nonverbal expressions of PR in his writings, Farber acknowledged that Rogers's nonverbal behaviors in his filmed interviews provided him (Farber) with a model for his own nonverbal expressions of care and support.

Over time, Carole's experience in treatment led to significant improvements. Her thinking became less black-and-white, and she developed an increased tolerance for uncertainty and ambiguity. As she began to view herself and others as amalgamations of strengths and weaknesses, her capacity to believe in her own value and to engage in intimate relationships improved. Carole also became better able to regulate her emotions, reducing the extent to which she experienced drama in her life. As her life and relationships improved, she began to accept herself to a far greater degree, "warts and all." Her self-deprecating comments became less frequent, and she began to more consistently experience pleasure in multiple areas of her life.

In working with Carole, Farber integrated elements from multiple psychotherapeutic approaches, including relationally oriented psychodynamic therapy, CBT, dialectical behavior therapy, and person-centered therapy. Having multiple ways to help individuals who suffer from the wounds of early intense trauma is, we believe, helpful. However, it was Carole who pointed out that above all, what touched her most profoundly in her treatment was the way her therapist consistently believed in her and supported her. While the case of Mary Jane illuminated the clinical improvements that emerged from a classic Rogerian approach that emphasized nondirectivity and acceptance (unconditional positive regard [UPR]), the case of Carole demonstrated the growth that can transpire when treatment is consistently infused with varied forms of PR.

POSITIVE REGARD AND PSYCHODYNAMIC PSYCHOTHERAPY: THE CASE OF TERRY WISE

Waking Up: Climbing Through the Darkness (Wise, 2012) is a compelling first-person account of the psychotherapy of a White woman, Terry Wise, who suffered from suicidal depression and substance abuse in her 30s following her husband's diagnosis and eventual death from amyotrophic lateral sclerosis (ALS). We learn, too, in this book that Terry's therapy needed to deal with her long-standing secrecy about the childhood sexual abuse she suffered. Terry's therapist was Dr. Betsy Glaser, a psychologist whose orientation was primarily psychodynamic but who, throughout this treatment, adopted aspects of multiple theoretical orientations. (Full disclosure as we recount this case: Betsy Glaser was a student of mine [BAF] several decades ago in the clinical psychology doctoral program within which I've served as a faculty member, and I've adopted this book as required reading for several graduate courses I teach. Betsy asked Terry to call her by her first name instead of "Doctor" early on in treatment, and, accordingly, we refer to Dr. Glaser by her first name throughout this account.)

Before this long-term course of treatment began, Terry had seen Betsy briefly to deal with the struggles of caring for her husband (Pete), who was dying of ALS. Betsy's empathy and compassion were already in evidence in this first treatment. She understood that Terry was under significant stress and encouraged her to take care of herself during the process of caring for Pete. At the last phase of Pete's life, Terry insisted that she was able to handle everything well, even as she was struggling mightily. Said Betsy, tenderly: "Oh Terry, just because you can physically do these things does not mean that you can do them psychologically" (Wise, 2012, p. 27). Although Terry had already dropped out of therapy by the time of Pete's death, Betsy sent a note of condolence and expressed her willingness to help. It was this note, according to Terry, that brought her back to therapy.

In their first session of this resumed therapy, Terry shared that her husband was diagnosed with this inevitably fatal illness just 3 weeks before their wedding. Betsy responded, "Gee, what incredible timing. I want to ask you again how I can be most helpful to you. It sounds like things must be really tough" (Wise, 2012, p. 18). Although we wouldn't ordinarily condone the sarcasm in the first phrase, there's nonetheless something empathic about it here—a sense of understanding the terrible absurdity and unfairness of life. Context plays a key role in the experience of PR, and because the pair had a previous, albeit short, history of prior treatment, and because Betsy was aware of how verbally sharp and intelligent Terry was—tellingly, she had been a successful attorney—Betsy likely understood that Terry would resonate with her choice of words. Moreover, this phrase was immediately followed by Betsy's invitation for Terry to voice her needs and ended with Betsy validating the difficulty of Terry's situation. This was not entirely a Rogerian response, to be sure, but the essential message in Betsy's words was infused with caring.

In this and subsequent sessions, Betsy encouraged Terry to explore the emotions that she was struggling with, suggesting that talking about her feelings would help her develop a better understanding of herself and ultimately help her cope with her understandable distress. However, she did not pressure Terry to disclose her more intense thoughts or feelings. Rather, when Terry expressed the fact that she was feeling emotionally overwhelmed, Betsy suggested that she should take her time to focus on any one issue that felt prominent and discussable. Again, this suggestion deviates from a classical Rogerian stance. Betsy is directive, voicing her opinion as to how Terry should best use her time in therapy. And yet, there is a sensitivity here that has a positively regarding feeling, something along the lines of "Although I am suggesting to you what I think would be most helpful to you, I will nonetheless respect your pace and your focus as we begin to explore these issues together."

As treatment proceeded, Terry acknowledged that she was resentful of her "strange" caretaking situation (i.e., near-total responsibility for her terminally ill husband). Betsy interrupted her to state, "That doesn't sound strange to me at all. I can see why you feel resentful" (Wise, 2012, p. 21). Rogers and other person-centered therapists would likely not interrupt, but we shouldn't lose sight of the empathy contained in the message itself: "I understand your feelings and fully accept them." One might even condone the interruption as a marker of how emphatically Betsy accepted her client's feelings about her situation. In addition, Betsy continued to assure Terry that self-care was essential and that she should not feel guilty for being unable to nurse her husband back to health. Drawing on a CBT approach, Betsy worked with Terry to change her narrative—from her sense that she was a "loser" to a self-perception that she was a quite likable human being with much to be proud of. To this end, she guided Terry to reflect on why many people in her life, including her husband and friends, loved her. Betsy reinforced this new narrative by disclosing her own warm and caring feelings toward Terry. In these matters, Betsy used a directive style that suited her and seemed appropriate to the clinical situation to demonstrate PR in the form of explicit affirmation of her client.

A surprise: Initially, Terry found Betsy's amicable and warm demeanor quite unappealing. Terry's sense was that her therapist was "a little too sickeningly sweet for my liking" (p. 18). This criticism is somewhat akin to the one that Rogers himself dealt with over the years—that his approach was too benign and superficial to effect any significant clinical change. Again, it may just be that the significant impact of a therapist's PR is experienced by clients only over time. That is, while the proximal effect of PR early in a client's treatment may result in a sense of "That's nice, but it doesn't get to the root of my problems or help me figure out what to do about them," over time, the cumulative effect of consistent PR is considerable, often leading to an increased sense of self-worth and agency that are important in their own right as well as allowing the client to better determine an effective course of action.

In fact, as therapy progressed, Terry's opinion about Betsy's style shifted dramatically: "Later, I learned that I had never been so wrong. It was a caring sweetness that partnered with a hard-line tenacity, but it was never in a sickening way" (Wise, 2012, p. 18). We cannot know the extent to which Betsy's PR, offered through consistent genuine care and liking, empathy, and explicit support, was instrumental in Terry's eventual healing. It is possible that the combination of traditionally conveyed PR (i.e., acceptance), explicitly affirming statements, and confrontation—what Terry deemed "tenacity"—is what made a difference. It is possible that other aspects of her treatment, including medications (antidepressants), made a difference. But all therapies contain multiple components that singly and in combination contribute to the variance in outcome. Whether as a main effect or part of an interaction term, it seems certain that PR, including its more explicit manifestations, played a significant role in Terry's successful therapeutic outcome.

As we've detailed, for some theorists and practitioners, therapist confrontation and challenge are legitimate aspects of an attitude of PR toward patients—if done sensitively and caringly. Betsy constantly prodded Terry to go deeper into her past and her feelings to understand her behavior and self-demeaning impulses. But even as she pushed, Betsy consistently channeled her inner Rogers and checked her understanding of what Terry was describing. Terry appreciated the value of Betsy's challenges, acknowledging that "it was an inroad to opening me up" (Wise, 2012, p. 28). And Betsy emphasized that while she might challenge Terry, she would never judge her—a very Rogerian (UPR) stance. There is nothing that you could say, Betsy communicated to her client, that would make me not like you (p. 100).

Betsy's way of challenging Terry to revisit her early painful narratives was infused with a great sense of sensitivity and caring:

> Terry, you are remembering things *today* with an *adult* mind. You are viewing your childhood with the incorporation of a lifetime of experiences, and what you *now* feel is right or wrong. Your mind was different when you were a child. If you work on recreating the context, we'll have a better understanding of what you knew and felt *at the time*. (Wise, 2012, p. 50)

When Terry continued to refuse to speak about her childhood, insisting that what she was going through now had nothing to do with earlier events in her life, Betsy's response was "I disagree, but okay. I want to respect your feelings about it" (Wise, 2012, p. 24). This was not quite nonjudgmental—Betsy was clearly offering a judgment—but as a compromise solution, it allowed for Terry to eventually speak about the abuse she suffered as a child, when she was ready to do so.

How else, other than the provision of empathy and support and the occasional challenge, did Betsy convey PR to her client? One way was by emphasizing to Terry how determined Betsy was to help Terry get better; in a related fashion, Betsy insisted that she would make herself available to Terry to the best of her ability. Indeed, she was quite flexible about the form of communication Terry might use to convey her thoughts and anxieties, including phone calls and email correspondence. Terry took great advantage of this unorthodox offer, often sending emails to Betsy; these provided much of the data for the book. Furthermore, Betsy used every opportunity she had to express to Terry that she wanted the best for her and would work with her to achieve Terry's goals: "I want our relationship to eventually free you, not bind you into one of dependent vulnerability" (Wise, 2012, p. 94).

Betsy's PR, mixed with a great deal of sincerity, manifested, too, as acceptance that the two of them would inevitably lose traction or feel disconnected or estranged at various points in the treatment. Such therapeutic ruptures (Safran & Muran, 2000) are often precipitated by a client's sense that the therapist has failed them in some way—that the therapist has, for example, missed a cue, been seemingly inattentive, confronted too harshly, or forgotten a critical detail. As a result, the relationship and therapeutic progress inevitably suffer. Betsy expressed these ideas to Terry as follows: "I will fail you in unknowing ways and I need you to talk to me and to trust [our relationship]" (Wise, 2012, p. 103). In this way, Betsy both reassured and affirmed to Terry—expressing confidence in Terry's ability to collaborate—that they could and would work together toward repairing ruptures when such occurred.

An example of their collaborative efforts to repair a rupture: Betsy became aware, via one of Terry's emails, that Terry was experiencing distress regarding their therapeutic relationship. Specifically, Terry had become very attached to Betsy and was torn by the realization that professional boundaries precluded some of the intimacy that Terry now craved. Terry longed to become an "insider" in her therapist's life, wanting Betsy to be both a mentor and a friend. This confession surprised Betsy, as she had not picked up on these feelings. In response, she wrote,

> I am so terribly sorry that I didn't pick up on the dilemma that has been tearing at you—wanting not to need or care, and yet needing and caring so profoundly that you are more scared than words can say. I've told you all along that I will screw up, and I did. (Wise, 2012, p. 94)

Her transparency, respect, empathy, and care for Terry in this communication are palpable. Betsy recognized the rupture in their relationship, named what was occurring in the moment, validated Terry's feelings, and repeatedly engaged in dialogue to help Terry understand that although she saw the boundaries as a roadblock between them, the boundaries actually served as "entrances" and "beginnings" to the possibilities and connections that could occur. But Betsy also understood the limits of interjecting herself into the therapy and the imperative to keep the focus on her client. Thus, reacting to her client's observation that she often displayed no more than a poker face in sessions, she replied, "If I started to emote the way I feel, the work would be about me and my feelings rather than about you" (Wise, 2012, p. 207).

PR, as research has shown, can include instances of tactful therapist disclosure. Reacting to Terry's acknowledgment of suicidal ideation, Betsy stated emphatically that she cared a great deal about Terry and that her death would impact her greatly: "Do you know how much I care about you? *I would have a hole in my heart forever if you died*" (Wise, 2012, p. 86). Terry was taken aback by her therapist's disclosure, having assumed that expressions of a therapist's true feelings were forbidden among mental health professionals. She later stated that Betsy's "availability and compassion" were "the most helpful words I could've heard that day," as they made her feel seen and cared for (p. 86).

And yet Terry did attempt suicide, taking what ordinarily would have been a lethal overdose of assorted pills. Miraculously, she survived. Often, when we think of individuals who have attempted or completed suicide, we feel sadness. But for those close to a suicidal individual, there is also a sense of betrayal. In the great (Oscar-winning) movie *Ordinary People*, the teenage protagonist (Conrad), who had made a serious suicide attempt, remarked to his therapist that "the mess" he had put his mother through was unforgivable (Redford, 1980). One chapter of *Waking Up: Climbing Through the Darkness* is titled "White Rage," a term that came directly from Betsy's description of what she felt in hearing the news of Terry's suicide attempt. Terry also understood the emotions she would stir in Betsy, before she attempted suicide:

> Would she despise me? I had promised her I would call her before I ever acted upon my desire to die, and she trusted me. There was no other way to interpret the statement I would be making. It was the ultimate "Fuck you." (Wise, 2012, p. 4)

And that was indeed how Betsy felt when she learned that Terry had attempted suicide. She felt Terry was deeming her inadequate—that her best efforts, including unflagging support and compassion, were just not enough for her. One effect of Betsy's rage was to revitalize Terry's awareness of just how much Betsy cared about her. Another consequence was for Betsy to insist that Terry promise to bring all of her pills into Betsy's office the next day. Betsy's insistence here, while again far too directive to align with Rogers's conceptualization of PR, certainly conveyed care ("I care about your life") and respect ("I respect you enough to repair this rupture").

Betsy's commitment to nondefensively acknowledge ruptures and collaboratively work toward repair is a form of PR evident throughout the full span of her work with Terry. For example, as Terry later showed signs of progress, and Betsy recommended reducing the frequency of their sessions, Terry registered a good deal of surprise and distress, fearing she was being forced to end therapy. Betsy quickly became aware that her well-meaning suggestion was not perceived as such by her client. She reassured Terry that she would not move toward termination until Terry felt herself ready to do so. Furthermore, Betsy emphasized that continuing their work would not at all feel burdensome to her "because when you care about someone there is no such thing as a quota" (Wise, 2012, p. 205).

Throughout this treatment, Betsy demonstrated that genuine care and challenge could coexist and perhaps even be mutually reinforcing. The PR that Betsy conveyed was not traditionally Rogerian. Betsy was often directive and sometimes judgmental; furthermore, the ways that she showed her care and support contained elements (e.g., confrontation) that Rogers would not have endorsed. But we believe that this expansive perspective on PR is more in accord with contemporary practitioners than is the PR provided by traditional person-centered therapists. In looking back on her successful treatment, Terry emphasized Betsy's PR—including, most prominently, her compassion, support, availability, and unwavering belief in the worth of her client.

POSITIVE REGARD AND CBT: THE CASE OF CHRISTINA

In some significant ways, person-centered therapy and CBT offer contrasting visions of psychotherapeutic treatment. Whereas the former emphasizes non-directionality, unconditional acceptance, and trust in clients' natural self-actualizing drive, the latter is a highly structured and often-manualized approach that targets and attempts to modify specific thoughts, feelings, and behaviors. Practitioners of the person-centered approach view the therapist–client relationship as the essential mutative ingredient in treatment; in contrast, CBT practitioners have, for the most part, touted their adherence to scientifically based principles of behavior change (e.g., learning theory) as the basis for their work. Furthermore, the practice of CBT therapists of disputing their clients' perceptions, including their self-evaluative statements and beliefs about others' intentions or meanings, can feel invalidating—quite the opposite of what person-centered therapists strive to convey. Despite such philosophical and practical differences, notable aspects of person-centered therapy, including the therapist's communication of PR, can be woven into the practice of CBT (Beck, 2011; Josefowitz & Myran, 2005). This should not be entirely surprising;

almost no therapeutic approach is entirely pure—rather, virtually all contain traces of other ways of practicing therapy. Rogers was occasionally interpretive; Freud was sometimes warm and overtly supportive. And most all contemporary psychotherapies have now come to believe in the fundamental importance of a good therapeutic relationship.

With these considerations in mind, we examined the ways in which Dr. Amy Wenzel (2016), in her video series, *Cognitive Behavioral Therapy Over Time*, established a therapeutic relationship with her client, one in which there were many notable instances of Rogers's facilitative conditions. In her introductory remarks, Dr. Wenzel provided a definition of CBT, noting that a cognitive behavioral therapist will "work with [their] clients to identify the manner in which they're interpreting and making meaning of their life circumstances to make sure they're viewing these circumstances in the most accurate and helpful way possible." Furthermore, she refuted the common myth that CBT focuses only on "surface level issues," with less emphasis on the therapeutic relationship than other modalities. She stated emphatically that these assumptions "really can't be further from the truth" and that there is a significant need for trust, empathy, and warmth in the cognitive behavioral relationship in order for treatment to be successful.

In Session 1, we were introduced to the client, a 25-year-old college student of Mexican-American descent named Christina.[1] Christina explained that she was struggling with feelings of immense responsibility and guilt as the primary caretaker for both her brother, who had cerebral palsy, and her mother, who was hearing impaired and suffered from cognitive disabilities. Although Christina's grandmother offered some assistance, Christina felt that the burden fell primarily on her to care for the family. As the client explained her situation, Dr. Wenzel responded empathically both verbally and physically, remaining attentive, nodding, leaning forward, and even grimacing when Christina recounted particularly difficult aspects of her daily life. After Christina finished sharing her narrative, Dr. Wenzel offered verbal reassurance in a soft, warm tone to her now-teary-eyed client: "If you can't have tears in a therapist's office, where can you have tears?" She went on to acknowledge that Christina was not necessarily viewing her external pressures in a distorted way and affirmed her client's sense that she had an immense amount of responsibility on her plate.

Dr. Wenzel explained to Christina that she wanted to focus equally on the development of a therapeutic relationship and on cognitive and behavioral change in their work and that it would be important to form a strong

---

[1]Some case aspects have been changed to protect client confidentiality.

personal connection within the dyad. As Christina continued to recount her situation, Dr. Wenzel frequently employed reflective listening techniques. In one instance, she validated Christina's perspective, stating, "You're saying something so important." She also asked her client, "Do you have the sense that it's your responsibility to provide?"—a question that seems to serve both as a means of checking the therapist's understanding and as an opportunity to offer an empathically tinged interpretation. In another instance, Dr. Wenzel employed this combination of reflective listening and interpretation as she said to Christina:

> Let me summarize so I make sure I'm understanding all this. You have this extremely complex family situation compared to other families, and it sounds like you were the caretaker and are very confident. You're carrying this tremendous— I don't want to call it a burden in a negative way—but sense that you need to be the provider. (Wenzel, 2016)

Christina responded in each case by confirming that Dr. Wenzel's understanding of the situation and its emotional implications was correct. She further acknowledged that Dr. Wenzel's approach—affirming her (Christina's) viewpoints and validating her experience—served as a relief to her and helped her feel sufficiently comfortable to continue the work.

Toward the middle of the session, Dr. Wenzel referred to the depression and anxiety questionnaires that Christina filled out prior to their meeting. Dr. Wenzel asked about coping mechanisms that Christina might use to combat the feelings of depression and anxiety that were indicated on the surveys. She also hypothesized that Christina might be partaking in "what the CDC [Centers for Disease Control and Prevention] would define as binge drinking" and suggested that Christina's sexual habits could be considered risky behaviors. Although these were not incorrect assumptions—indeed, Christina later confirmed that these behaviors may be problematic—it is noteworthy that the client was not the one to draw attention to any of these issues. It was Dr. Wenzel who both brought them up and deemed them maladaptive behaviors that should be addressed in treatment, an approach that we would surely not see in a person-centered therapy. While many of Dr. Wenzel's questions and statements validated Christina's perspectives and were infused with a sense of empathy and caring, Christina was nonetheless being evaluated: Her risky behaviors had been deemed necessary targets of change.

As the sessions progressed, a format began to emerge. Dr. Wenzel would first take stock of Christina's depression and anxiety surveys, briefly discussing events that happened over the past weeks and then discussing the week's homework. While several external factors in Christina's life were "intensifying," she stated that she had experienced Dr. Wenzel's "openness

[as] concrete and informative," acknowledging that learning that her experience "isn't too unique" comforted her and gave her a sense that she could get better. As they dove into Christina's continued frustrations, Dr. Wenzel empathized with and complimented her, saying,

> I get that you're stuck, but I want you to give yourself some credit. You have accomplished some amazing things given your life circumstances, so I think there is already a core of strength and resiliency here. We're just going to figure out how to harness that and make it work for you.

Dr. Wenzel's PR here, in the form of explicit compliments, was likely especially meaningful to Christina, who often struggled with feeling "less than."

As the dyad discussed Christina's past week, we developed a strong sense that Dr. Wenzel truly cared about her client and wanted to be helpful and supportive but that she would also be quite directive and even somewhat judgmental. Unlike Rogers, she would not accept without comment all of Christina's behavioral choices or affective states. When Christina expressed the sense that she was overwhelmed by her family responsibilities, Dr. Wenzel suggested they do some problem solving around Christina's many responsibilities and recommended using a thought record. This approach seemed to pull Christina out of her despair for a moment and was likely reassuring inasmuch as Dr. Wenzel was providing hope in the form of a solution. However, this intervention also short-circuited Christina's expression of her feelings and, per Rogers, seemed to imply that Christina was incapable of discovering solutions on her own.

When Christina expressed a desire to strengthen her relationship with her mother, Dr. Wenzel appeared acutely attuned, saying,

> I'm seeing through the tears in your eyes that it is even more important here how you build a relationship with your mom. . . . What if we were to brainstorm ways to connect with her more in a way that you maximize the time you do have together? . . . I don't think your mom expects you to really be there all the time.

Christina responded that she was relieved, feeling that things were more "doable and organized," and Dr. Wenzel reassured her that "there is no right or wrong. This is an experience you are owning."

In Session 3, Christina stated that she had a particularly hard week with regard to familial conflict, but she noted, too, that the exercises were beginning to enable her to pinpoint her triggers and cope in more productive ways. When Dr. Wenzel asked what was different that week, Christina responded that she was too broke to drink or smoke but that she also wanted to be stronger. Dr. Wenzel remarked that this was a notable change from other weeks and then explicitly affirmed Christina: "Coming here was a really big step in facing this, and now that you and I are facing this work together you're really gathering that strength that you always had inside."

While Christina continued to appear frustrated with herself for getting upset and having negative thoughts, Dr. Wenzel was increasingly reassuring, stating that "some of those statements are really powerful, and most people if they truly believed those things would feel really badly as well." Dr. Wenzel then introduced the idea of "thinking traps," or flawed automatic thoughts, taking her client through a list of common traps (e.g., "all or nothing thinking" and "jumping to conclusions") and encouraging her to choose the ones that resonated most with her. In stating, "You've said you wanted a way to organize your thoughts—this will be a way of doing that," Dr. Wenzel showed she had heard, and was attentive to, Christina's needs. Even when she was directive in her leading of the session, Dr. Wenzel typically posed her responses to Christina either as references to things the client had said previously, as in the aforementioned example, or as a question, beginning with "I wonder if" or "Do you think?" This seemed to soften her directivity and provide Christina room within which to correct Dr. Wenzel or steer the session in a slightly different direction. Additionally, in response to one of Christina's harshest convictions—the belief that she was stupid—Dr. Wenzel offered a deeply affirming counterpoint:

> I can tell you from my point of view you are absolutely not stupid. You've gone through some really incredible life experiences and you're still in the thick of it, so it makes a lot of sense that because of these past experiences you would view the world in a certain way.

Dr. Wenzel's ability to offer Christina a revised and meaningful way to understand her perceived weakness was yet another powerful form of PR offered and, in line with our research, the therapist-provided behavior clients consider to be most affirming (see Chapter 6). As such, and despite the challenging undertones, we suspect that Rogers would approve.

The same format and trends continued in subsequent sessions. In Session 4, Christina continued to score lower on the depression and anxiety scales, even in light of her having been in a car accident and having a panic attack requiring hospitalization between sessions. In this session, much of the focus was on Christina's feeling that she deserved the bad things that happened to her. Dr. Wenzel encouraged her to challenge these thoughts, asking Christina to "tell [her] some of the reasons why you're worthy. Tell me about the lives you've touched." Christina brought up two friends she supported through self-harm and suicidal ideation, and Dr. Wenzel encouraged her to continue, admonishing her not to "disqualify the positive" and going on to draw Christina's attention to her care for her family, commitment to her education, love of dance and music, and overall good citizenship, ultimately concluding with the observation "It sounds like there are some things you want to change, but you are a worthy person." Dr. Wenzel was consistently affirming of Christina's progress in this session and, more generally, became increasingly complimentary and positively regarding throughout their work together. Her explicit support and validation challenged Christina's negative self-talk, while also showing Dr. Wenzel's commitment to the therapeutic relationship. These kinds of statements, which may have come off as disingenuous in earlier sessions, now proved equal parts nurturing, personalized, and authentic, illustrating that an intuitive sense of timing can be a key consideration in offering particular forms of PR.

The final two sessions followed a similar arc and dealt primarily with Christina's thinking traps, especially her sense that she was "stupid." Dr. Wenzel was consistently affirming, stating, "You've had 23 years of thinking in this way, I actually think you're making tremendous progress" and "It will take a while to forge a new pathway in your brain." We see this reframing echoed in Christina's own sentiments, as she began to take the therapist's reassurance and affirmations to heart, even using similar words to acknowledge that she should be more patient with herself and that change would take time. Dr. Wenzel continued to validate Christina's perspective while offering positive reframes of her negative self-statements: "I think anybody in your situation would feel this way," "You really did your brother a good service . . . what a gift you're giving him," and "That definitely shows me that you're a worthy person." In these comments, Dr. Wenzel appeared to give Christina the permission to trust herself and acknowledge her needs in a way that neither she nor her family members had been able to provide in the past. One can see the seeds of unconditional positive self-regard being planted throughout the session.

The final session culminated in Christina stating that this work had led to a clearer sense of herself and the ability to refrain from victimizing herself. The pair discussed, in depth, the progress Christina had made with respect to the goals she set out in the beginning of treatment and made a plan for Christina's continuing therapy with a new practitioner, with whom Dr. Wenzel said she would be happy to talk about the work they had completed so far. With her characteristic warmth, Dr. Wenzel expressed to Christina, "This may be the end of our face-to-face work, but I do hope we keep in touch. I wish you the best of luck with everything."

In this case of a client who presented with immense feelings of hopelessness and despair, Dr. Wenzel's basic CBT approach was suffused with consistent warmth, empathy, reassurances of worth, and explicit affirmations. This was surely not a person-centered therapy, but it did contain significant elements of this approach, providing a fine example of how Rogers's core conditions, including PR, may be manifest in a treatment not typically known or assumed to be conducive to his ideas.

Ideally, these examples would have reflected greater client and therapist diversity. All clients were female, in their 20s or 30s; all of the therapists were White. Still, taken together, these four real-life clinical vignettes illustrate the multiple ways that PR can be conveyed within and across a variety of psychotherapeutic approaches. At times, these positively regarding behaviors and statements seem part of an ongoing flow of dialogue, simply the way that a caring, accepting, responsive therapist naturally interacts with their valued client. PR here seems contextual, a near-constant, predictable climate within the therapeutic relationship. This was what Rogers essentially had in mind— that PR is a pervasive attitude, not a discrete intervention or technique. But at other times in these clinical summaries, the therapist's PR seems prominent within the dialogue, an exclamation point of sorts, a means of accentuating a particular moment or client statement. At these times, PR moves from background to foreground, approximating—as with Rogers's communication to Gloria, in their taped demonstration interview, that she looked like a pretty nice daughter (see Chapter 3)—the feel of a corrective emotional experience. These are moments when PR leads to a more intense-than-usual emotional connection and/or a greater acceptance and appreciation of oneself. There are in-between points, as well, on this hypothetical continuum—PR statements or behaviors that, while not quite attaining the status of a corrective emotional experience, are nevertheless experienced by the client as especially meaningful or moving.

Another takeaway from these vignettes: Communicating PR to a client, even on a steady basis, does not radically alter the nature of a therapist's preferred theoretical stance or clinical style. The provision of PR can feel seamless in a person-centered therapy, in a primarily psychodynamic therapy, in an eclectic psychotherapy, and even in a CBT treatment. If it does not, per Rogers, inevitably lead to treatment success when paired with empathy and congruence, it surely enhances the development and maintenance of an effective therapeutic relationship and facilitates the therapist's ability to effectively employ other therapeutic tools associated with the therapist's primary theoretical orientation. These are undoubtedly significant and important achievements in themselves.

In Chapter 9, the concluding chapter of this book, we examine the controversies and criticisms that have beset the concept of PR since its early formulation by Rogers, draw some conclusions about its place in psychotherapeutic treatment, and offer some recommendations for training and practice.

9 POSITIVE REGARD AND PSYCHOTHERAPY

Controversies, Criticisms, and Conclusions

The greatest happiness of life is the conviction that we are loved, loved for ourselves—say rather, loved in spite of ourselves.

—Victor Hugo, *Les Misérables*

Although the foundational importance of the psychotherapy relationship is now recognized by virtually all forms of contemporary psychotherapy, all aspects of the relationship are not equally accepted. Generally speaking, the need for a strong therapeutic alliance is universally acknowledged, whereas the same cannot be said for positive regard (PR), at least not in its original nonjudgmental acceptance (unconditional positive regard [UPR]) form. In this final chapter, we review the controversies and criticisms surrounding the concept of PR, provide suggestions for future research in this area and recommendations for training, and derive some conclusions about the place of PR within a broad spectrum of psychotherapies. What we strive to emphasize throughout is that although we find some criticisms of the boundaries and traditionally defining features of PR (especially its UPR branch) to be valid, we nevertheless believe strongly in its

https://doi.org/10.1037/0000312-010
Understanding and Enhancing Positive Regard in Psychotherapy: Carl Rogers and Beyond, by B. A. Farber, J. Y. Suzuki, and D. Ort

essential value as one component of a comprehensive treatment strategy. No brand of psychotherapy and no psychotherapeutic concept is immune from criticism. Each is more than likely to have its limitations. As our understanding and use of PR evolve as a result of both clinical innovation and research findings—trends consistent with the history of most aspects of psychotherapy—we hope that even greater numbers of practitioners will appreciate its value in helping clients move toward growth and healing.

CONTROVERSIES AND CRITICISMS

The great majority of criticisms leveled at PR are not focused on the legitimacy or importance of the concept, especially in its more extended, liberal form. That is, those criticizing aspects of PR tend to basically concur with the overall idea that it is vital for clients to perceive their therapist's acceptance and support, even if they contest the degree to which and methods by which this should occur. The controversies and criticisms have thus centered on several issues, most persistently the contention that, contrary to the UPR premise, a therapist cannot be invariantly nonjudgmental and accepting of all that clients feel, think, do, or intend to do. Other questions and criticisms have been posed, including those related to the breadth by which PR should be defined, the possibility that it inhibits change, and the extent to which it can effect change. For each of these issues, we first present the nature of the criticism and then offer alternative—and, in our estimation, balanced—perspectives on the arguments raised.

The Criticism: Positive Regard Cannot and Should Not Be Unconditional

We begin by focusing on the issue of the presumed incompatibility of a therapist's nonjudgmental attitude and that therapist's genuine feelings and values. Indeed, this was the issue that Rogers was most often confronted with in his career. Per the recollection of Dale Larson, one of his colleagues, Rogers was often challenged, at conferences, with questions of the following sort: "Your client says he is going to murder all White or Black people and you don't feel revulsed and judgmental?" Rogers typically responded with a "deep within there is goodness" kind of response, one that felt inadequate to many (D. Larson, personal communication, October 10, 2020).

In fact, multiple theorists have contended that PR cannot be unconditionally conveyed by a therapist. Lietaer (2001) observed: "Both within and without client-centered therapy this basic attitude [unconditional acceptance] has not always been welcomed in an unconditionally positive way" (p. 91).

In fact, Lietaer placed some of the blame for this state of affairs on Rogers himself, suggesting that Rogers did not sufficiently elaborate on what he meant by unconditional acceptance or sufficiently attend to its problematic features. The belief that PR, either as UPR or as broader-based variable, is inevitably conditional tends to be based on the proposition that all therapists selectively affirm and attune to certain client statements to the exclusion of others. Therapists' feelings about their clients and the concerns both are struggling with—what psychodynamic therapists deem countertransference—necessarily affect their ability to be fully accepting and supportive of their clients. Moreover, the understandable press to effect positive changes in clients' lives limits a therapist's ability to be nondirective and unconditionally regarding.

One form of directivity and selectivity was acknowledged by Rogers: that he was interested primarily in client feelings or experience and often attempted to shift the therapeutic narrative to clients' felt meanings—to what is now often termed "lived experience." Rogers (1970) wrote about this intention in describing his work with an encounter group:

> There is no doubt that I am selective in my listening, hence "directive" if people wish to accuse me of this. I am centered in the group member who is speaking, and am unquestionably much less interested in the details of his quarrel with his wife, or of his difficulties on the job, or his disagreement with what has just been said, than in the *meaning* these experiences have for him now and the *feelings* they arouse in him. It is to these meanings and feelings that I try to respond. (pp. 50–51)

Rogers's aim, then, was to accept every client feeling, whatever the content of that feeling, and his attention and empathy tended to be in the service of focusing on and exploring deeply what his client experienced in the moment.

But, like all of us, Rogers had his blind spots and was uneven in what he accepted in others. The late existential psychologist Rollo May (1982) averred that Rogers and his colleagues were unwilling to acknowledge or accept the *daimonic* in others—the universal human need to assert one's individuality. As a consequence, according to May, client-centered therapists are unable to deal with their clients' hostile and aggressive feelings. Although not quite accepting the validity of May's criticism, Rogers (1970) acknowledged, "I find it difficult to be easily or quickly aware of angry feelings in myself. I deplore this; am slowly learning in this respect" (p. 54).

That therapists cannot be unconditional in their acceptance is also based on a related proposition: that certain client behaviors cannot or should not be accepted or supported. Implicitly accepting or more actively affirming such behaviors may violate one's own moral values and inadvertently serve to perpetuate undesirable actions. As Hendricks (2001) phrased it: "How do I prize and feel warmly towards someone who is repetitively angry, stuck, depressed, cannot process his feelings, and attacks me for not changing him?" (p. 127). A variation on these two propositions is that there is a fundamental disjunction between a therapist's attempts to be unconditionally regarding and that therapist's attempts to be genuine in interactions with clients.

How, then, has the person-centered community responded to this set of criticisms? Most commonly, theorists have argued that acceptance within the context of PR should be understood in terms of acceptance of clients' feelings or experience rather than acceptance or support of their behaviors. Lietaer (2001), who has written extensively about this issue, expressed this very view:

> My client ought to experience the freedom to feel *anything* with me; he should sense that I am open to his experience and will not judge it. . . . [However], this attitude of receptivity toward the inner experiential world of my client does not mean that I welcome all behavior equally. Both within and without the relationship there can be specific behaviors of which I disapprove, would like to change, or simply do not accept. (p. 92)

Lietaer's (2001) stance, one echoed by many of the therapists in our study (see Chapter 7, this volume), was that one need not and should not approve of a client's racist feelings or inappropriate, narcissistic, or dysfunctional behavior but, rather, work to understand—empathically and nonjudgmentally—the roots of such feelings and behavior. "Without approving of it, I accept his behavior as something that is there 'for the time being' and go with him into the personal problems that lie behind it" (Lietaer, 2001, p. 92). The position articulated here—consistent with the psychodynamic focus on understanding the genesis of problematic behavioral patterns—is also somewhat akin to parents who convey the message to a child that while the child will always be loved, some behaviors are not going to be met with absolute acceptance.

Moreover, noted Lietaer (2001), if a client wants or needs something that feels inappropriate from the therapeutic relationship itself—for example, a friendship or a sexual relationship—the therapist can still accept the feelings or needs while concomitantly conveying the message that although everything can be discussed, not everything can be allowed:

> It remains important that she [a client] can express and discuss everything that she experiences with respect to me, without my becoming reluctant or rejecting her as a person; but with regard to her behavior, I do confront her with my limits. (p. 92)

There is an overlap here with the psychoanalytic notion of "benevolent neutrality." For example, Kernberg (1976), an eminent psychoanalytic thinker, described the neutrality of the analyst in terms of their concerns for those with whom they work, an attitude that protects patients' autonomy, independence, and capacity to accomplish their work on their own. Substitute "positive regard of the counselor" in this sentence for "neutrality of the analyst," and it would be easy to believe that Rogers himself had written it.

Thus, for Lietaer, invariant acceptance of the person and nonacceptance of certain behaviors can comfortably coexist. Other person-centered theorists have expressed similar views. For example, according to Mearns and Thorne (2007),

> The client feels that the counselor values him consistently throughout the relationship, despite the fact that he may not value himself and even if the counselor does not approve of all the client's behavior. It is possible to accept the client while still not liking some of the things he does. (p. 96)

Cain (2010) took an even more liberal position in terms of the boundaries of the therapist's PR, suggesting that clients do not expect their therapists to unconditionally accept all their behaviors, thoughts, and feelings. Rather, he stated, clients need only to feel that they will not be "rejected or abandoned despite their therapists' dislike or disapproval of some attitudes, feelings, values, or behavior" (p. 39). Moreover, contended Cain, if therapists were truly unconditional in their acceptance, they could not possibly be entirely genuine and, as a result, would seem less trustworthy to clients.

The question, then, of how PR is possible in the face of difficult or onerous client behaviors can be answered in two different, albeit related, ways. For Rogers, the task was to find and affirm the inevitable goodness that lies beneath the manifest difficult behaviors. But most theorists acknowledge, in one way or another, that PR is not and cannot be truly unconditional. That is, there are true limits to the degree to which this can occur, limits that most clients accept and may even benefit from. From this perspective—one with which we fully concur—therapists are "allowed" to experience disapproval as long as they convey a primary attitude of acceptance and support.

The Criticism: Conveying Positive Regard May Reinforce Clients' Old Patterns and Defenses

If clients perceive consistent PR from a therapist, along with accompanying attitudes of empathy and genuineness, they may indeed grow psychologically— or, in the words of Carl Rogers, become more fully actualized. But there's another scenario that Rogers did not consider: that in the absence of challenge, confrontation, or active questioning, clients may remain stuck. The argument here is that therapists whose conceptions of PR don't allow them to push or encourage change or to challenge clients to take risks, but rather solely affirm or nonjudgmentally accept their clients' feelings, thoughts, or behavior, are inadvertently colluding with a patient's defenses, conveying a message of approval of the status quo. In another context, that of discussing the challenges of writing fiction, Klein (2021) pointed to the tension "between empathizing with others and holding them to account." The hypothesis—or, rather, pointed suggestion—in regard to person-centered therapy is that some therapists operating within this modality cannot sufficiently distance themselves from a reflexively accepting stance that at times fails to serve the needs of their clients.

A variation on this critique is that there is too great a potential for patients to assume and expect PR in the absence of change or in the continued presence of dysfunctional behavior. Again, such an occurrence could reinforce behaviors that clients themselves would like to change. The therapist's PR here might work in the service of clients' ambivalence around actual change, allowing them to persevere with chronic resistant or defensive patterns. Dale Larson (personal communication, October 10, 2020) suggested that this was where Carl Rogers could himself get stuck—that he did not have a model for disrupting clients' dysfunctional interpersonal cycles, such as Wachtel (2008, 2014) proposed.

In her book *Maybe You Should Talk to Someone: A Therapist, Her Therapist, and Our Lives Revealed*, Gottlieb (2019) addressed how PR can go wrong or be misunderstood by clients: "Therapists will be supportive, but our support is for your growth, not for your low opinion of your partner. (Our role is to understand your perspective but not necessarily to endorse it)" (p. 124). Gottlieb's observations here strike us as entirely accurate. Clients are often looking to their therapists for affirmation of their strongly held opinions and feelings, and it may be easy for therapists to fall into this trap. Even "hmm hmm" or attempts at empathy—"You really were so very angry"—may give a client the impression that their therapist agrees with the expressed sentiment.

These overlapping critiques of PR essentially suggest that its conveyance in the absence of some attitude or intervention that counters an unwavering acceptance of all that clients present in sessions is clinically problematic. We believe that there is some truth to this contention, but we also believe that it needs to be seen with a far broader lens. Any intervention or attitude, singularly or indiscriminately applied, is likely to be clinically problematic, whether it is communicating PR, offering psychoanalytic interpretations, reframing narratives, or disputing irrational beliefs. We also contend that refraining from judgment and holding steadfastly to an accepting stance are difficult clinical tasks. In the popular Netflix series *The Crown*, Queen Mary (played by Eileen Atkins) has the following to say about the burdens of neutrality: "To be impartial is not natural, not human" (Morgan & Jarrold, 2016). We believe that there is a place for explicit affirmations and/or gentle challenges within a broad understanding of PR; we also believe that there is a place for acceptance without judgment or appraisal.

THE ARGUMENT: POSITIVE REGARD IS NOT INEVITABLY HELPFUL AND MAY EVEN BE COUNTERPRODUCTIVE

To be sure, Rogers did not suggest that by itself, the therapist's communication of PR would lead to patient growth; rather, he contended that this attitude along with the other facilitative conditions are the necessary and sufficient conditions for client change (Rogers, 1957). But there is a clear assumption in his writings, and those of other person-centered therapists, that PR is an invariably beneficial clinical attitude.

In contrast, there is an emerging sense that less-than-optimal consequences of PR are real possibilities in some cases and under certain circumstances. For example, Gelso (2019) noted a way in which PR—at least, that type of PR that includes explicit affirmation—can work against the best interest of the client: "Direct expressions of loving feelings by the therapist may be experienced as oppressive by the patient, and may actually inhibit the patient's expression of negative feelings toward the therapist" (p. 133). Gelso's thoughts here seem clinically astute and provide some additional nuance to research findings (Farber, Blanchard, & Love, 2019) that indicate that clients struggle mightily with disclosing their honest feelings about therapy and the therapeutic relationship. For some clients, a therapist's consistently affirming and caring attitude may add a layer of burden to the existing difficulty of letting their therapist know their true feelings. This may take the form of client thought such as "My therapist cares so much about me, I just can't disappoint her with my sense that this therapy is not what I want and that I need more from her than she's providing."

A therapist's PR may also feel patronizing, or even undeserved, to some clients. In this regard, Agnes Callard, a philosopher and college professor, wrote an opinion piece in *The New York Times* about her conflict in letting others know about what she called "The Events." Based on her somewhat cryptic description, it seems that she was abused at some point in her life. The specific nature of her conflict lies in her apprehension about how others might react to this experience; she is especially averse to the specter of others voicing their appreciation for her courage in coming forward with her story:

> I don't want you to think you know the meaning of The Events; I don't want to be classified as damaged; I don't want you to feel good about yourself for believing me; I don't want you to feel sorry for me; and most of all, I don't want you to praise my courage for "coming forward" or for "surviving." The prospect of receiving praise or honor for this revelation fills me with rage—when I imagine your admiration, I immediately imagine throwing it back in your face. (Callard, 2020, para. 5)

The point is that clients vary significantly in the extent to which they can accept their therapist's relational stance as deeply infused with PR. Like Callard, there are groups of clients for whom explicitly conveyed PR may feel troubling or burdensome. For some, PR may feel like a means for their therapists to elicit some form of PR (e.g., affirmation) for themselves. For example, for clients who have had narcissistic parents or partners, the experience of being cared for has typically meant that they are expected to reciprocate in kind. This client's internal dialogue might be along the lines of "I'm not really deserving of all this support—I'm a troubled, difficult person. What does my therapist want or expect in return?" Similarly, consistently provided PR can result in some clients trying too hard to be compliant, to be "good" in order to continue receiving their therapists' warmth and acceptance. In particular, clients with anxiety disorders may become more anxious when positively regarded. They get hooked on it, and when it is not forthcoming, their symptoms may intensify. Patients diagnosed with borderline personality disorder may also react less than positively to their therapist's PR. Prunetti et al. (2008) provided evidence that therapists' validation is often disorganizing to this group of patients. Following validation (as defined by Linehan), these patients' responses revealed significantly higher rates of temporary metacognitive failure—an inability to think coherently about their own thoughts—in comparison to responses elicited by neutral, nonvalidating interventions.

Writing well before the advent of client- or person-centered therapy, Freud (1923) anticipated these types of clinical reactions to a therapist's PR, reactions he attributed to unconscious guilt:

> There are certain people who behave in a quite peculiar fashion during the work of analysis. When one speaks hopefully to them or expresses satisfaction with the progress of the treatment, they show signs of discontent and their condition invariably becomes worse. . . . One becomes convinced, not only that such people cannot endure any praise or appreciation, but that they react inversely to the progress of the treatment. (p. 49)

More generally, affirmation can feel less than respectful to clients if not complemented with honest, constructive feedback. Without accurate feedback from their therapist, clients may, paradoxically, feel less seen, less understood, and less confident in their therapist's abilities. Even when the positive feedback is accurate, clients with toxic or negative self-views may struggle in much the same way. An excellent example of this comes from Tara Westover's (2018) book, *Educated: A Memoir*. Here, the author responded to her experience of being praised by a professor who noted that her essay was one of the best he had read in 30 years:

> I was prepared for insults but not for this. . . . I could tolerate any form of cruelty better than kindness. Praise was a poison to me; I choked on it. I wanted the

professor to shout at me, wanted it so deeply I felt dizzy from the deprivation. The ugliness of me had to be given expression. (p. 240)

In a similar vein, Rogers (1951) restated the words of a client, Miss Cam:

Say something unpleasant about me, and I'd agree immediately and wholeheartedly, but try to tell me something nice about myself, and I'd spend hours trying to convince you, to explain in great detail how wrong you were. It wasn't false modesty either, I really felt desperately uncomfortable and dishonest in accepting appreciation. (p. 110)

Despite these protestations, Miss Cam's work with her client-centered therapist ultimately seemed to be helpful. At the conclusion of her therapy, she reported, "I can see that things aren't hopeless, that it is in me, and that I can do something about it" (Rogers, 1951, p. 126).

Thus, for some clients, PR is not invariably helpful and may even have paradoxical consequences. We regard this, however, as inevitable. As we've previously noted, no single clinical intervention or attitude (or medication, for that matter) will prove beneficial to all individuals. Moreover, Rogers never claimed that PR alone would be sufficient in improving clients' lives. We remain convinced that it is helpful in most cases, especially in combination with other clinical means and when its allowable features are expanded to meet the needs of individual clients.

The Criticism: The Therapist's Positive Regard Should Not Be Restricted to What Rogers Advocated

The classic position, emanating from the writings of Rogers, is that PR should essentially be communicated to clients as acceptance, nonjudgment, warmth, and caring. Most would agree that these are commendable and often-effective means of connecting with and enabling clients to feel understood and supported. But herein lies a potential problem, one we've noted throughout these chapters: Restricting the expressions of PR to the ways in which Rogers and like-minded others have suggested leaves out the possibility that—for some clients, at least some of the time—PR can best be expressed and have the most robust clinical effects through the therapist's constructive feedback, challenges, narrative reformulation, or compliments. Stated otherwise, PR may be best communicated not within its typically delimited forms (as "acceptance" or even "warm acceptance") but rather through consideration of individual client needs. For example, in Miss Cam's case (see the previous section), there might have been added value to the therapy had Rogers's communication of PR— once he sensed she was better able to tolerate it—included explicit affirmations, encouragement, or offering Miss Cam new ways of understanding and accepting parts of herself that she viewed as weaknesses.

The counterargument here is that whereas challenge, compliments, words of reassurance, and the like are sometimes helpful clinical interventions, they should not be considered within the legitimate domain of PR. That is, by including these kinds of statements into our notions of PR, we change too radically the essence of what Rogers meant by it, such that it is no longer significantly defined by the quality of nonjudgmental acceptance. There is certainly some legitimacy to this perspective; altering some basic elements of a concept renders it something else. Nevertheless, there are two primary reasons why we believe that, on balance, modifying the terms or definition of PR is more legitimate than otherwise. The first is that, as indicated in earlier chapters, therapists as well as clients overwhelmingly endorse multiple, highly potent ways for the therapist to communicate PR, whether defined in research protocols in terms of "affirmation" or "validation," or more broadly, in terms of interest, acceptance, respect, care, and liking. To reiterate: Many of these items, including those that speak to the therapist's explicit words of support and direct attempts to help clients accept more benign narratives about their lives, go well beyond traditional conceptualizations of PR. Our own research (see Chapter 6) suggests strongly that clients see their therapists' "flexible responsiveness" as a core component of PR. Different clients may need different forms of PR to heal their wounded selves; each client may need different forms of PR at different moments of therapy. In this regard, Gelso (2019) offered the following:

> It is important to be thoughtful about when to support a given patient, and in what way. Some patients do indeed need the therapist's support (e.g., advice, structuring, explicit statements of caring), and might move backwards without it. On the other hand, most do best when the therapist adopts a more neutral stance (with some deviations along the way), so long as the neutrality is in a context of empathy, caring, and affirmation. (p. 149)

Moreover, even those therapists who essentially adhere to traditional views about the ways that PR should be communicated may interject something into their communication to clients that deviates from the assumptions of Rogers. Rogers himself tells Gloria (his demonstration interview client) that he thinks she looks like a pretty nice daughter (see Chapter 3). Wilkins (2000/2001), among the strongest advocates for positioning PR as *the* essential ingredient in client change, offered an example of using PR with a difficult patient that seemingly includes a psychodynamic element. The example he offered was in the context of explaining why providing PR to some patients is difficult but nevertheless possible: "As I listened and responded to him, I began to wonder about what life experiences had led him to his extreme [racist, misogynistic] views" (p. 40). One size of PR seemingly does not fit all clients, an assumption consistent with the more general adage that every client deserves a unique brand of therapy.

The second reason for believing that reconceptualizing the bounds of PR is appropriate and necessary lies in Rogers's (1959) assumption about what PR actually remediates. His belief was that many individuals have been subject to conditions of worth in childhood that damaged their sense of self, a supposition that has been supported by empirical research on the enduring emotional consequences of parental conditional regard (e.g., Roth et al., 2009). According to Rogers, such individuals are in need of PR as a condition for their healing. What PR is said to do is to unleash the actualizing tendency, the inherent movement toward growth in all humans. Bozarth (1998) provided an excellent summation of this position:

> It is the actualizing tendency that is the fundamental curative factor lying within the person. The reference to unconditional positive regard as the curative factor assumes the thwarting of the natural tendency: hence, making it necessary that the client becomes more deeply connected with the actualizing tendency through unconditional positive self-regard. (p. 82)

If the primary aim of PR is to invigorate the actualizing tendency, in turn ameliorating the psychic damage done by early conditions of worth, then the following question needs to be asked: What type of PR best accomplishes this process? Again, for Rogers, the answer here is the therapist's consistent displays of acceptance and caring, often communicated through empathic responsiveness. There is, however, no evidence that this classic form of PR is any more or less effective in attenuating early psychological injuries or generating psychological growth than a host of other types of support or affirmations. The Rogerian way of expressing PR may even be the most productive, universal, and enduring way of catalyzing tendencies toward growth. However, some clients may need different means to foster their growth. PR, even with great doses of empathy, may just not be enough for some clients to move toward their potential. As Wilkins (2000/2001) noted,

> If it is accepted that psychopathological and/or antisocial ways of being are induced by conditions of worth, and that unconditional positive regard is a way of redressing these, then it is implicit that effective therapy is limited only by the therapist's ability to experience and convey this attitude to the client. (pp. 42–43)

Many, though certainly not all, theorists and clinicians within the person-centered world have come to this more flexible position—and, based on the research we have conducted, we concur.

The Criticism: Positive Regard Has Only a Modest Association With Clinical Outcome

Consistent with Rogers's theory, PR has proven to be significantly associated with therapeutic change. However, meta-analyses have reported only a modest association between PR and outcome. And whereas it can be argued that the dependent variable in most empirical outcome studies—symptom relief—is inconsistent with the tenets of person-centered therapy (which, as noted earlier, privileges self-regard and self-actualization), there still exists a problem: Person-centered therapy and humanistic therapy of any sort (or, for that matter, psychodynamic therapies) tend not to explicitly provide clients with answers, solutions, or coping strategies that are surely needed for some disorders. Patients with borderline personality disorder, for example, need specific help with the coping mechanisms and emotion regulation strategies they lack; PR, even in combination with the other facilitative conditions, is unlikely to provide them with the skills to negotiate stressful situations or the vicissitudes of interpersonal relationships. Patients diagnosed with obsessive–compulsive disorder are unlikely to be helped by PR (or insight, for that matter); they need to be taught to gradually tolerate stimuli (e.g., germ-contaminated doorknobs) they experience as toxic. The point is that acceptance, nonjudgment, and warmth—even when paired with empathy and therapist genuineness—cannot substitute for the skills some clients lack.

Assuming a broader perspective, though, all individual therapist, client, and system variables tend to account for relatively small parts of the process–outcome equation (e.g., Lambert, 2013; Norcross, 2002, 2011; Norcross & Lambert, 2019). Moreover, relational elements, taken collectively, account for the greatest degree of variance in outcome (Wampold & Imel, 2015). In short, that PR is limited in its healing potential does not make it insignificant. That in some or perhaps many instances it cannot by itself, or even in combination with the other facilitative conditions, effect all-encompassing clinical changes does not lessen its important, often-foundational role in the process of most every psychotherapeutic approach.

FUTURE RESEARCH DIRECTIONS

As therapies have become more relationally oriented, clinical and research efforts to identify and evaluate the components of effective therapeutic relationships have increased. We have noted in earlier chapters some of the research done on the association of PR to outcome and on client and therapist perceptions of the most frequently conveyed and most potent forms of PR. Clearly, though, many questions remain to be answered about the nature and consequences of PR in psychotherapy. Among the most salient unanswered or understudied questions are the following:

- How consistent is the communication of PR, both within and across therapists? Do therapists tend to maintain a steady dose of PR to individual clients? To what extent do therapists vary their provision of PR across clients? How extensive is the variation of PR across therapists? As Norcross and Lambert (2019) have shown, "effective psychotherapists responsively provide varying levels of relationship elements in different cases and, within the same case, at different moments" (p. 312).

- What therapist, client, or process variables contribute to the variability in therapist-provided PR? Some of our own qualitative studies have begun to offer preliminary answers to this question, analyzing how issues of client and therapist identity (e.g., race, ethnicity, gender, sexual orientation, country of origin) may affect the provision of PR (see especially Chapters 6 and 7), but many of these putative factors are likely to be interactive in ways that only quantitative large-scale studies with sufficient power can identify. Furthermore, other factors, including client and therapist attachment style, may affect the variability of PR—and these have not been studied.

- How do temporal factors affect both the communication and receipt of PR? Perhaps clients habituate to their therapists' expression of PR, necessitating "larger" doses over time, or perhaps some clients who are initially averse to expressions of PR become better able to receive it over time. Perhaps, too, PR, especially in the form of nonjudgmental acceptance, changes in the later stages of long-term treatments. As the therapist's caring and investment in effective treatment increase over time, they may be tempted to provide direct advice or clinical suggestions for the "good" of the client. More generally, do certain phases of treatment (e.g., the beginning phase, the termination phase) or certain occurrences in treatment (e.g., alliance ruptures) require special consideration in how therapists provide PR?

- What kinds of clients (i.e., with what diagnoses and/or personality styles) are most likely to benefit most from therapists' overall provision of PR? Similarly, which forms of PR are most effective with which clients? As noted earlier (see Chapter 3), Eckert et al. (1988) found that of the four components they hypothesized compose PR—warmth, respect, acceptance, and interest—warmth and respect were most responsible for symptom change among clients with the most severe symptoms. This was a study of only 77 clients, and each of these assumed components was assessed via a single question; moreover, no follow-up research has confirmed these results.

Nevertheless, it is a provocative finding, suggestive of the possibility that different forms of PR (as in Eckert et al., 1988) or different clusters (warmth/authenticity, flexible responsiveness, empathic acceptance, as per our findings noted in Chapter 6) are most effective with different types of clients. Data have begun to answer this general question (see Chapters 6 and 7), but studies with larger and more diverse samples are needed.

- What are the proximal and distal effects of confronting and/or challenging clients in the context of providing more traditional means of communicating PR? Can occasional confrontations and/or challenges intensify the potency of an otherwise traditionally communicated attitude of PR? As Orlinsky and Howard (1986) observed, "Normally, this [affirmation] is experienced as warmth and acceptance, but there are occasions when genuine caring leads to confrontation and challenge" (p. 348). But little is known about the specific ways of being challenging or confrontational that are most likely to feel positively regarding to clients.

- How is PR most often conveyed in other-than individual therapy with adult clients? For example, how does PR change when therapists are working with children? The meta-analyses we performed on the relation of PR to outcome (Farber, Suzuki, & Lynch, 2019) revealed only a small number of studies ($n = 11$) that looked at this specific association. Similarly, research is needed to investigate how PR is most typically and/or effectively conveyed in couples, family, or group therapy. What are the effects of providing PR to an individual within a therapeutic modality that involves multiple clients, as when working with couples, families, or groups? In a related vein, it would be instructive to investigate how PR is communicated most typically and effectively in 12-step programs. Does the effectiveness of PR increase exponentially when offered by multiple individuals in an essentially leaderless group? And how does the provision of PR change in settings other than traditional clinical settings? For example, are there normative, if different, patterns of PR in forensic settings?

- How does the provision of PR change when the therapist has lived experience with the disorder targeted by the treatment? Do those who have experienced a specific disorder (e.g., an eating disorder, substance abuse) become more or less positively regarding—and if so, in what ways—when working with others with such disorders? And do clients perceive the PR of such individuals as being especially potent?

- How does providing PR to one's clients affect the therapist? Does it have an influence on the therapist's sense of self? On their relationships with others? Does conveying PR with high frequency in therapy inhibit or facilitate the expression of PR in other contexts?

- And a final question, one that reflects the changing nature of psychotherapy: How is PR conveyed and received differently in newer forms of therapy, including teletherapy and text-based applications, including those that rely on artificial intelligence? Emerging research has indicated that the association between the therapeutic alliance and treatment outcome in internet-based psychotherapy is equivalent to that in face-to-face psychotherapy (Flückiger et al., 2018) and that clients generally perceive their therapists to be *more* positively regarding in the context of teletherapy than in in-person therapy (Ort & Farber, 2021). However, given the burgeoning use of teletherapy and newer forms of text-based applications, far more research is needed to ascertain clients' and therapists' perceptions of PR over the course of these types of treatment.

Many of these questions could be summarized by appropriating the oft-cited psychotherapy specificity question (Paul, 1967): What kinds of PR, offered to what kinds of patients, by what kinds of therapists, at what moments in therapy, in what clinical settings, lead to what kinds of immediate and cumulative effects?

IMPLICATIONS FOR TRAINING AND PRACTICE

Our recommendations for training and practice rest on converging aspects of theory and research. First, the results of recent meta-analyses have indicated a significant association between therapists' adoption of positively regarding behaviors and good clinical outcome, for virtually all therapists across all theoretical models at all levels of experience and with most all types of clients. Although there are small exceptions to these general findings, including indications (some from Rogers himself) that more severely disturbed clients are more resistant to the mutative effects of PR, the overall and consistent empirical evidence points to the value of therapists adopting an attitude of PR toward their clients. Second, the writings of notable theorists within the person-centered community (see Chapter 3), as well as the results of our own work on the constituent elements of PR (see Chapters 6 and 7), suggest that therapists' PR can be conveyed and received in a multifaceted manner.

Taken together, these findings suggest that students should be taught the value of and means toward adopting a positively regarding attitude toward clients. The extant clinical and research data also indicate that students should learn more about Rogers's facilitative conditions in general. Thus, we believe that students should read primary source material—that is, a good deal of Carl Rogers's writing. In particular, we would suggest Kirschenbaum and Henderson's edited volume, *The Carl Rogers Reader* (Rogers, 1989); *Client-Centered Therapy: Its Current Practice, Implications, and Theory* (Rogers, 1951); *On Becoming a Person: A Therapist's View of Psychotherapy* (Rogers, 1961); *A Way of Being* (Rogers, 1980); and *The Psychotherapy of Carl Rogers: Cases and Commentary* (Farber et al., 1996). We also suggest Cain's (2010) overview of the recent state of the person-centered movement, *Person-Centered Psychotherapies*.

We believe that including Rogers's writings on the facilitative conditions of psychotherapy would contribute greatly to every beginning practicum in graduate training programs, regardless of the theoretical orientation of that course. We suggest, too, that practicum instructors remind students that practices that encourage therapists to approach patients through a lens of detachment and neutrality—or through exclusively dispassionate, technically driven interventions—are contraindicated by research evidence pointing strongly to the importance of relational considerations in effecting positive clinical outcome. And, in this regard, we strongly suggest that students become knowledgeable about the burgeoning clinical and research work on a multitude of relational variables, including but not limited to Rogers's facilitative conditions. The current best book in this area is the recent two-volume edition of *Psychotherapy Relationships That Work* (Norcross & Lambert, 2019; Norcross & Wampold, 2019), with chapters on such relational variables as the therapeutic alliance, attachment style, cultural adaptations and multicultural competence, and client preferences. We also highly recommend Hill's (2020) *Helping Skills: Facilitating Exploration, Insight, and Action*, with an entire chapter on "skills for providing support" that includes helpful illustrative material on how best to listen and support clients via nonverbal, paraverbal, and verbal behaviors, as well as how best to incorporate cultural considerations into one's listening and support.

What may be obvious but nevertheless worth noting: Viewing Rogers's 30-minute demonstration session with Gloria is not enough. We imagine that many students' knowledge of Rogers begins and ends with seeing this film. It is a perfectly good introduction to Rogers's work and therapeutic philosophy. "All in all," Rogers said in his postinterview musings that are part of the film (Shostrom, 1965), "I feel good about this interview." But we believe, too, that solely on the basis of viewing this film, many students are left with the wrong impression of what an overall attitude of PR truly entails. My (BAF) sense in showing this film many times over many years is that burgeoning clinicians have a tendency to reduce Rogers's pervasive acceptance of a person's feelings and experience, including the "deeper core of the person" (Lietaer, 1984, p. 47), to the rendering of a heartfelt compliment (e.g., "You look to me like a pretty nice daughter") or even the adoption of a "nice person" attitude. Watching multiple videos of Rogers's work, reading summaries or transcripts of his sessions, observing others who have implemented similar concepts into their practice (e.g., Linehan, 2006), and reviewing research and theory that speak to the possibilities of conveying PR in nontraditional ways (e.g., Bozarth & Wilkins, 2001; Farber & Ort, 2021; Suzuki & Farber, 2016) are all likely to greatly expand students' understanding of the importance and implications of adopting this attitude into their clinical work.

We also believe in the value of clinical supervisors monitoring the quality and consistency of PR that supervisees offer their clients. Although this may be partially accomplished through supervisory discussions of countertransference (i.e., of therapists' emotional attitudes toward patients), our suggestion here is for supervisors to focus, at least occasionally, on the specific ways in which trainees' acceptance, liking, caring, and affirmation of their clients have been conveyed (or not) in sessions and what the clinical consequences of these actions have been. As many pundits have remarked, the truth—and perhaps the devil, too—is in the details. We believe that supervisors would do well to find out how and why their supervisees convey certain positively regarding attitudes and adopt certain words and phrases but omit others and how clients have reacted to different manifestations of this general attitude. In this vein, too, supervisors might inquire as to whether their supervisees still hold negative views of being positively regarding to clients or of any of Rogers's facilitative conditions, views that might link support or PR to superficiality. Whereas that strikes us as an unfortunate possibility, it would also hardly be surprising: More than a few mentors (and supervisors) of therapists-in-training likely have biases, based on their own training, such that they continue to perceive person-centered therapy or any of its fundamental practices as insufficiently "deep," effective, or empirically supported.

We believe, too, that supervisors, to the extent that they themselves value the place of PR in therapy, should inquire as to how adopting a positively regarding attitude, or specific ways of doing so, has affected their super-visees' professional self-image and the ways in which they conceptualize their developing theoretical model. Most supervisors, regardless of their theoretical orientation, are likely to endorse without reservation the value of empathy and perhaps other relational variables (e.g., identifying and resolving rupture alliances). The evidence suggests strongly that endorsing multiple ways of making clients feel supported, cared for, and affirmed contributes to therapeutic success, an outcome that in turn contributes to beginning therapists' sense of self-efficacy and professional confidence.

Many of the recommendations supporting the value of including the consistent communication of PR within therapists' overall relational stance are as true for experienced therapists as they are for those in training. In summarizing the research done on the association of relational variables to clinical outcome, Norcross and Lambert's (2018) first practice recommendation was that practitioners should prioritize the development and maintenance of the therapy relationship and especially attend to those "relationship elements found to be demonstrably and probably effective" (p. 309). PR is, in fact, one of the elements in the "demonstrably effective" category—as is empathy. (Based on the research evidence, congruence was categorized as "probably effective"). Thus, therapists of all types, including those who prioritize empirically supported interventions, should feel empowered and legitimized to include communicating PR to their clients.

Another of Norcross and Lambert's (2018) conclusions was that adapting evidence-based relational elements to specific patient characteristics—what the authors deem the "whole person" (p. 309)—enhances the effectiveness of treatment. Thus, practitioners should give themselves permission to be flexible in conveying relational elements in their efforts to be optimally effective. There is no one best way of being positively regarding or empathic or establishing an effective therapeutic alliance. Characteristics and needs of specific patients are clearly paramount to consider. Some patients will benefit more from a more-or-less nonjudgmental, accepting stance, whereas others will seem to need greater explicit reinforcement (affirmations) in order to try out new feelings or behaviors. Moreover, as is true of so many other therapeutic considerations, the exact nature of how one provides relational elements to clients is dependent on multiple factors. Therapists at all levels of experience and adherent to all types of theoretical models should feel free to adapt their provision of relational elements in accord with their own style and patient needs. Although in some ways PR will look and feel the same when offered by a person-centered therapist as when offered by a cognitive behavior therapy practitioner, in other ways, this cannot be entirely true. One's values and beliefs necessarily affect one's way of questioning, affirming, accepting, or challenging patients: "Techniques are embedded in a specific and ever changing relationship, and . . . the relationship is altered by virtue of the techniques employed" (K. Benau, personal communication, January 17, 2021).

CONCLUSION

PR is an important clinical component, a significant piece of the outcome equation—perhaps especially so for healthier clients. However, by itself or even in combination with Roger's other core conditions, therapist provision of PR is no panacea—as no therapeutic variable is. Better, we are suggesting, to regard PR as clinically valuable, perhaps even necessary in some cases, a foundational piece that—along with other common factors (e.g., empathy, genuineness, collaboration and goal consensus, responsiveness, feedback, repairing alliance ruptures) and other specific therapeutic interventions, including interpretations, narrative reframing, cognitive restructuring, and emotion processing—generates new client thoughts, feelings, and behavior, including increases in client disclosure and self-esteem.

We contend, too, and have consistently suggested as much in these pages, that PR can and should be communicated in multiple ways, responsive to the changing needs of each client. Therapist responsiveness to clients' needs for PR tends to be constrained by bias and/or strict adherence to theoretical principles. As Wilkins (2000/2001) wisely noted, "Dogma is the enemy of unconditional positive regard" (p. 35). And, we would add, the enemy of PR (the omnibus version), as well. There is, we believe, a place for variable forms of PR within and across therapy cases, though the heuristics for determining which forms of PR are best suited for which types of client problems or characteristics have yet to be established. This, of course, is true not just for PR but for virtually every relational variable. We are also aware of the conceptual problem with overextending the domain of what can be considered PR. If every intervention or attitude that leads to clients feeling affirmed, supported, cared about, or well respected is included within the category of PR, the term itself loses meaning. We believe there must be some consistent bases of therapist-provided empathy, acceptance, warmth, and support that define the boundaries of PR—and yet, we also believe there are some in-the-moment exceptions (e.g., confrontations) that don't rest easily within this general definition.

One way of partially resolving this dilemma is by conceptualizing PR as both an enduring climate or attitude of acceptance and an intervention that may take multiple and sometimes paradoxical forms. Even as a therapist maintains a resolute attitude of overall acceptance and essential nonjudgment, they may sometimes need to modify the ways this attitude is manifest, even combining it, at times, with behaviors (e.g., challenge) that may seem antithetical to Rogerian ideas. Saying to a client, "I believe you can do this" has elements of both support and gentle challenge. But that PR is hard to define or operationalize should not be surprising: Its "cousin," empathy, is said to have at least 43 different definitions (Cuff et al., 2016).

Our sense is that the consistent communication of PR to clients—and, even more so, the consistent communication of the unconditional acceptance aspect of PR—should be regarded as ideals. Therapists will inevitably fall short, but what is important, what will be sensed and internalized by the client, is the therapist's aspiration to be consistently accepting, supportive, and responsive to individual needs and preferences: "This is someone, a highly respected and valued someone, who is always trying to understand what I'm thinking and feeling, who believes in me, supports me, cares about me, wants me to believe in myself." This is what we believe stays with a client and makes a difference.

PR is a relative outlier within Rogers's facilitative conditions. Since the late 1990s, there has been a great resurgence of research into empathy, helping to "re-legitimize empathy as a central element of psychotherapy" (Elliott et al., 2018, p. 400). Concomitantly, there has been a renewed interest in the concept of therapist authenticity, expressed in the writings of contemporary relationally oriented therapists (e.g., Aron, 1996; Gelso et al., 2019; McWilliams, 2004; Wachtel, 2008) and in the research and theoretical literature on therapist disclosure (e.g., Henretty & Levitt, 2010; Knox & Hill, 2003; Kolden et al., 2019). Compared with supervisory-reinforced efforts as to how to best communicate empathy and allow their authentic selves in their clinical work, our sense is that beginning therapists are often on their own in making decisions about how and when to best convey an attitude of PR with their clients. We regard this as another significant reason to include the study of PR in all mental health training programs. Beginning therapists—indeed all therapists—are likely to be positively regarding to their clients but may not feel sufficiently empowered to maintain or develop their skill in communicating this attitude and its associated behaviors.

Finally, we believe that the study of PR is especially important in these troubled and divisive times. Beset by political, economic, health, and environmental crises, so many therapy clients come to treatment feeling exhausted, distracted, overloaded, unsure of themselves and their future. A 2018 Cigna survey (Polack, 2018) of over 20,000 adults in the United States found that 46% of respondents *always* or *sometimes* felt alone, and 47% *sometimes* or *always* felt left out; 27% *never* or *rarely* felt there were people who understood them. A similar 2019 Cigna (2020) survey of over 10,000 adults in the United States found that 61% reported that they were *lonely*. And both of these surveys were conducted before the global COVID-19 pandemic.

These are difficult times, and so many individuals—clients of psychotherapy or otherwise—are feeling disconnected and alone. There are fewer opportunities now, circa 2022, to be truly heard, attended to, accepted, respected, and affirmed. A few months before this book went to press, David Brooks (2021), a columnist for *The New York Times*, wrote a piece in which he opined about the characteristics of wisdom in a divisive "ideological age." Although no psychologist was cited, the title of the article, "Wisdom Isn't What You Think It Is," as well as its contents, was vintage Carl Rogers. Brooks wrote:

> When wisdom has shown up in my life, it's been less a body of knowledge and more a way of interacting, less the dropping of secret information, more a way of relating that helped me stumble to my own realizations. . . . Wise people don't tell us what to do, they start by witnessing our story. (paras. 5, 7)

Brooks used the phrase "unconditional positive regard" to speak to the "quality of attention" he suggested was at the heart of wisdom.

The idea, developed and popularized by Carl Rogers, that there are those who want to know us, hear our story, and understand us deeply and who—despite all that they have learned—accept us, affirm us, and believe fully in our ability to grow speaks to what is likely a universal need. This dynamic is powerful in all interpersonal relations but has special resonance in psychotherapy, given the status and authority bestowed on the therapist. We hope that this message, this idea, will grow to be an even more fully accepted and integral aspect of all psychotherapies in ways that best benefit all psychotherapy clients.

References

Antheunis, M. L., Schouten, A. P., Valkenburg, P. M., & Peter, J. (2012). Interactive uncertainty reduction strategies and verbal affection in computer-mediated communication. *Communication Research*, *39*(6), 757–780. https://doi.org/10.1177/0093650211410420

Aron, L. (1996). *A meeting of minds: Mutuality in psychoanalysis*. The Analytic Press.

Baima, T., & Sude, M. E. (2020). What White mental health professionals need to understand about Whiteness: A Delphi study. *Journal of Marital and Family Therapy*, *46*(1), 62–80. https://doi.org/10.1111/jmft.12385

Baldwin, M. (2000). Interview with Carl Rogers on the use of the self in therapy. In M. Baldwin (Ed.), *The use of self in therapy* (2nd ed., pp. 29–38). Haworth Press.

Barrett-Lennard, G. T. (1962). Dimensions of therapist response as causal factors in therapeutic change. *Psychological Monographs: General and Applied*, *76*(43), 1–36. https://doi.org/10.1037/h0093918

Barrett-Lennard, G. T. (1964). *The relationship inventory. Form OS-M-64 and OS-F-64, Form MO-M-64 and MO-F-64*. University of New England.

Barrett-Lennard, G. T. (1978). The relationship inventory: Later development and adaptations. *JSAS Catalog of Selected Documents in Psychology*, *8*(68).

Barrett-Lennard, G. T. (1986). The relationship inventory now: Issues and advances in theory, method, and use. In L. S. Greenberg & W. M. Pinsof (Eds.), *The psychotherapeutic process: A research handbook* (pp. 439–476). Guilford Press.

Barrett-Lennard, G. T. (2015). *The relationship inventory: A complete resource and guide*. John Wiley & Sons.

Bauman, G. (2001). Unconditional positive regard. In J. D. Bozarth & P. Wilkins (Eds.), *Rogers' therapeutic conditions: Evolution, theory and practice: Vol. 3. Unconditional positive regard* (pp. 3–4). PCCS Books.

Baym, N. K. (2010). *Personal connections in the digital age*. Polity Press.

Beck, A. T. (1979). *Cognitive therapy and the emotional disorders*. Penguin.

Beck, J. S. (2011). *Cognitive behavior therapy: Basics and beyond* (2nd ed.). Guilford Press.

Becker, E. (1973). *The denial of death*. Free Press.

Ben-Eliyahu, A., Yoviene Sykes, L. A., & Rhodes, J. E. (2021). Someone who 'gets' me: Adolescents' perceptions of positive regard from natural mentors. *Mentoring & Tutoring, 29*(3), 1–23. https://doi.org/10.1080/13611267.2021.1927438

Benjamin, L. S. (1984). Principles of prediction using structural analysis of social behavior (SASB). In R. A. Zucker, J. Aronoff, & A. J. Rabin (Eds.), *Personality and the prediction of behavior* (pp. 121–173). Academic Press.

Bergin, A. E., & Garfield, S. L. (Eds.). (1971). *Handbook of psychotherapy and behavior change: An empirical analysis*. John Wiley & Sons.

Bergin, A. E., & Garfield, S. L. (Eds.). (1993). *Handbook of psychotherapy and behavior change* (4th ed.). John Wiley & Sons.

Bohart, A. C. (2015). From there and back again. *Journal of Clinical Psychology, 71*(11), 1060–1069. https://doi.org/10.1002/jclp.22216

Bohart, A. C. (2020, June). *Notes on positive regard* [Paper presentation]. Society for Psychotherapy Research 51st International Annual Meeting, Amherst, MA, United States.

Bohart, A. C., & Greenberg, L. S. (Eds.). (1997). *Empathy reconsidered: New directions in psychotherapy*. American Psychological Association. https://doi.org/10.1037/10226-000

Bologna, C. (2019, May 31). *35 hilarious tweets about therapy*. HuffPost. https://www.huffpost.com/entry/tweets-seeing-a-therapist_l_5cdb27e9e4b0790953dec08c

Bond, C. F., Jr., & DePaulo, B. M. (2006). Accuracy of deception judgments. *Personality and Social Psychology Review, 10*(3), 214–234. https://doi.org/10.1207/s15327957pspr1003_2

Bowlby, J. (1951). *Maternal care & mental health*. World Health Organization Monograph Series.

Bowlby, J. (1977). The making and breaking of affectional bonds: I. Aetiology and psychopathology in the light of attachment theory. *The British Journal of Psychiatry, 130*(3), 201–210. https://doi.org/10.1192/bjp.130.3.201

Bowlby, J. (1988). *A secure base: Parent–child attachment and healthy human development*. Basic Books.

Bozarth, J. (2001). Client-centered unconditional positive regard: A historical perspective. In J. Bozarth & P. Wilkins (Eds.), *Rogers' therapeutic conditions: Evolution, theory and practice: Vol. 3. Unconditional positive regard* (pp. 5–18). PCCS Books.

Bozarth, J., & Wilkins, P. (Eds.). (2001). *Rogers' therapeutic conditions: Evolution, theory and practice: Vol. 3. Unconditional positive regard*. PCCS Books.

Bozarth, J. D. (1996). A theoretical reconsideration of the necessary and sufficient conditions for therapeutic personality change. *The Person-Centered Journal, 3*(1), 44–51. https://adpca.org/wp-content/uploads/2020/11/Bozarth-Therapeutic-PCJ-3_1.pdf

Bozarth, J. D. (1998). *Person-centered therapy: A revolutionary paradigm*. PCCS Books.

Bozarth, J. D. (2013). Unconditional positive regard. In M. Cooper, M. O'Hara, P. F. Schmid, & A. C. Bohart (Eds.), *The handbook of person-centred psychotherapy and counselling* (2nd ed., pp. 180–192). Palgrave Macmillan/Springer Nature. https://doi.org/10.1007/978-1-137-32900-4_12

Breger, L. (2009). *A dream of undying fame: How Freud betrayed his mentor and invented psychoanalysis*. Basic Books.

Brodley, B. T., & Bradburn, W. M. (2015). Did Carl Rogers' positive view of human nature bias his psychotherapy? *The Person Centered Journal, 22*(1-2), 81–112. https://adpca.org/wp-content/uploads/2020/12/22_5.pdf

Brodley, B. T., & Schneider, C. (2001). Unconditional positive regard as communicated through verbal behavior in client-centered therapy. In J. D. Bozarth & P. Wilkins (Eds.), *Rogers' therapeutic conditions: Evolution, theory and practice: Vol. 3. Unconditional positive regard* (pp. 156–172). PCCS Books.

Brooks, A. C. (2019, March 2). Our culture of contempt. *The New York Times*. https://www.nytimes.com/2019/03/02/opinion/sunday/political-polarization.html

Brooks, D. (2021, April 15). Wisdom isn't what you think it is. *The New York Times*. https://www.nytimes.com/2021/04/15/opinion/wisdom-attention-listening.html

Buber, M. (1937). *I and thou*. T. & T. Clark.

Burns, D. D., & Nolen-Hoeksema, S. (1992). Therapeutic empathy and recovery from depression in cognitive-behavioral therapy: A structural equation model. *Journal of Consulting and Clinical Psychology, 60*(3), 441–449. https://doi.org/10.1037/0022-006X.60.3.441

Cain, D. J. (2010). *Person-centered psychotherapies*. American Psychological Association.

Callard, A. (2020, November 30). I don't want you to 'believe' me. I want you to listen. *The New York Times*. https://www.nytimes.com/2020/11/30/opinion/i-dont-want-you-to-believe-me-i-want-you-to-listen.html

Carnegie, D. (1936). *How to win friends and influence people*. Simon & Schuster.

Casemore, R., & Tudway, J. (2012). *Person-centred therapy and CBT: Siblings not rivals*. SAGE.

Castonguay, L. G., & Hill, C. E. (Eds.). (2012). *Transformation in psychotherapy: Corrective experiences across cognitive behavioral, humanistic, and psychodynamic approaches*. American Psychological Association. https://doi.org/10.1037/13747-000

Castonguay, L. G., Youn, S. J., Xiao, H., & McAleavey, A. A. (2018). The therapeutic relationship: A warm, important, and potentially mutative factor in cognitive-behavioral therapy. In O. Tishby & H. Wiseman (Eds.), *Developing the therapeutic relationship: Integrating case studies, research, and practice* (pp. 157–179). American Psychological Association. https://doi.org/10.1037/0000093-008

Christakis, N. A. (2019). *Blueprint: The evolutionary origins of a good society*. Little, Brown Spark.

Christchurch shooting survivor says he forgives his wife's killer [Video file]. (2019, March 17). BBC News. https://www.bbc.com/news/av/world-asia-47602781

Cigna. (2020). *Loneliness is at epidemic levels in America.* https://www.cigna.com/about-us/newsroom/studies-and-reports/combatting-loneliness/

Clemence, A. J., Hilsenroth, M. J., Ackerman, S. J., Strassle, C. G., & Handler, L. (2005). Facets of the therapeutic alliance and perceived progress in psychotherapy: Relationship between patient and therapist perspectives. *Clinical Psychology & Psychotherapy: An International Journal of Theory & Practice, 12*(6), 443–454. https://doi.org/10.1002/cpp.467

Cook, J. M., Biyanova, T., & Coyne, J. C. (2009). Influential psychotherapy figures, authors, and books: An Internet survey of over 2,000 psychotherapists. *Psychotherapy: Theory, Research, Practice, Training, 46*(1), 42–51. https://doi.org/10.1037/a0015152

Cooper, M., O'Hara, M., Schmid, P. F., & Bohart, A. C. (Eds.). (2013). *The handbook of person-centred psychotherapy and counselling* (2nd ed.). Palgrave Macmillan/Springer Nature. https://doi.org/10.1007/978-1-137-32900-4

Cramer, D. (1986). An item factor analysis of the revised Barrett-Lennard Relationship Inventory. *British Journal of Guidance & Counselling, 14*(3), 314–325. https://doi.org/10.1080/03069888608253521

Cuff, B. M. P., Brown, S. J., Taylor, L., & Howat, D. J. (2016). Empathy: A review of the concept. *Emotion Review, 8*(2), 144–153. https://doi.org/10.1177/1754073914558466

Curtis, R., Field, C., Knaan-Kostman, I., & Mannix, K. (2004). What 75 psychoanalysts found helpful and hurtful in their own analyses. *Psychoanalytic Psychology, 21*(2), 183–202. https://doi.org/10.1037/0736-9735.21.2.183

Derks, D., Fischer, A. H., & Bos, A. E. R. (2008). The role of emotion in computer-mediated communication: A review. *Computers in Human Behavior, 24*(3), 766–785. https://doi.org/10.1016/j.chb.2007.04.004

Dewey, J. (1939). Theory of valuation. *International encyclopedia of unified science.* University of Chicago Press.

DuBois, W. E. B. (2019). *The souls of Black folk essays and sketches.* G & D Media. (Original work published 1903)

Eckert, P. A., Abeles, N., & Graham, R. N. (1988). Symptom severity, psychotherapy process, and outcome. *Professional Psychology: Research and Practice, 19*(5), 560–564. https://doi.org/10.1037/0735-7028.19.5.560

Elliott, R., Bohart, A. C., Watson, J. C., & Murphy, D. (2018). Therapist empathy and client outcome: An updated meta-analysis. *Psychotherapy, 55*(4), 399–410. https://doi.org/10.1037/pst0000175

Elliott, R., Bohart, A. C., Watson, J. C., & Murphy, D. (2019). Empathy. In J. C. Norcross & M. J. Lambert (Eds.), *Psychotherapy relationships that work: Vol. 1. Evidence-based therapist contributions* (3rd ed., pp. 245–287). Oxford University Press.

Elliott, R., & Farber, B. A. (2010). Carl Rogers: Idealistic pragmatist and psychotherapy research pioneer. In L. G. Castonguay, J. C. Muran, L. Angus, J. A. Hayes,

N. Ladany, & T. Anderson (Eds.), *Bringing psychotherapy research to life: Understanding change through the work of leading clinical researchers* (pp. 17–27). American Psychological Association. https://doi.org/10.1037/12137-002

Eysenck, H. J. (1952). The effects of psychotherapy: An evaluation. *Journal of Consulting Psychology, 16*(5), 319–324. https://doi.org/10.1037/h0063633

Eysenck, H. J. (1966). *The effects of psychotherapy*. International Science Press.

Farber, B. A. (2006). *Self-disclosure in psychotherapy*. Guilford Press.

Farber, B. A. (2007). On the enduring and substantial influence of Carl Rogers' not-quite necessary nor sufficient conditions. *Psychotherapy: Theory, Research, Practice, Training, 44*(3), 289–294. https://doi.org/10.1037/0033-3204.44.3.289

Farber, B. A., Blanchard, M., & Love, M. (2019). *Secrets and lies in psychotherapy*. American Psychological Association. https://doi.org/10.1037/0000128-000

Farber, B. A., Bohart, A. C., & Stiles, W. B. (2012). Corrective (emotional) experience in person-centered therapy: Carl Rogers and Gloria Redux. In L. G. Castonguay & C. E. Hill (Eds.), *Transformation in psychotherapy: Corrective experiences across cognitive behavioral, humanistic, and psychodynamic approaches* (pp. 103–119). American Psychological Association. https://doi.org/10.1037/13747-007

Farber, B. A., Brink, D. C., & Raskin, P. M. (Eds.). (1996). *The psychotherapy of Carl Rogers: Cases and commentary*. Guilford Press.

Farber, B. A., & Doolin, E. M. (2011). Positive regard and affirmation. In J. C. Norcross (Ed.), *Psychotherapy relationships that work: Evidence-based responsiveness* (2nd ed., pp. 168–186). Oxford University Press. https://doi.org/10.1093/acprof:oso/9780199737208.003.0008

Farber, B. A., & Lane, J. S. (2002). Positive regard. In J. C. Norcross (Ed.), *Psychotherapy relationships that work: Therapist contributions and responsiveness to patients* (pp. 175–194). Oxford University Press.

Farber, B. A., Lippert, R., & Nevas, D. (1995). The therapist as attachment figure. *Psychotherapy, 32*(2), 204–212. https://doi.org/10.1037/0033-3204.32.2.204

Farber, B. A., & Metzger, J. A. (2009). The therapist as secure base. In J. H. Obegi & E. Berant (Eds.), *Attachment theory and research in clinical work with adults* (pp. 46–70). Guilford Press.

Farber, B. A., & Ort, D. (2021, June 23–26). *Therapists' attitudes regarding the communication of positive regard* [Paper presentation]. Society for Psychotherapy Research Annual Meeting, Heidelberg, Germany.

Farber, B. A., & Suzuki, J. Y. (2018). Affirming the case for positive regard. In O. Tishby & H. Wiseman (Eds.), *Developing the therapeutic relationship: Integrating case studies, research, and practice* (pp. 211–233). American Psychological Association. https://doi.org/10.1037/0000093-010

Farber, B. A., Suzuki, J. Y., & Lynch, D. A. (2019). Positive regard and affirmation. In J. C. Norcross & M. J. Lambert (Eds.), *Psychotherapy relationships that work: Vol. 1. Evidence-based therapist contributions* (3rd ed., pp. 288–322). Oxford University Press. https://doi.org/10.1093/med-psych/9780190843953.003.0008

Fehr, S. S. (2003). *Introduction to group therapy: A practical guide* (2nd ed.). Routledge.

Feijt, M., de Kort, Y., Bongers, I., Bierbooms, J., Westerink, J., & IJsselsteijn, W. (2020). Mental health care goes online: Practitioners' experiences of providing mental health care during the COVID-19 pandemic. *Cyberpsychology, Behavior, and Social Networking, 23*(12), 860–864. https://doi.org/10.1089/cyber.2020.0370

Flückiger, C., Del Re, A. C., Wampold, B. E., & Horvath, A. O. (2018). The alliance in adult psychotherapy: A meta-analytic synthesis. *Psychotherapy, 55*(4), 316–340. https://doi.org/10.1037/pst0000172

Frank, J. D. (1961). *On persuasion and healing: A comparative study of psychotherapy*. Johns Hopkins University Press.

The Fred Rogers Company. (2018). *About Fred Rogers*. https://www.misterrogers.org/about-fred-rogers/

Freire, E. (2001). Unconditional positive regard: The distinctive feature of client-centred therapy. In J. D. Bozarth & P. Wilkins (Eds.), *Rogers' therapeutic conditions: Evolution, theory and practice: Vol. 3. Unconditional positive regard* (pp. 145–155). PCCS Books.

Freire, E., Koller, S. H., Piason, A., & da Silva, R. B. (2005). Person-centered therapy with impoverished, maltreated, and neglected children and adolescents in Brazil. *Journal of Mental Health Counseling, 27*(3), 225–237. https://doi.org/10.17744/mehc.27.3.6p6qm84wqkkxp2a5

Freud, S. (1923). The ego and the id. In J. Strachey (Ed.), *The standard edition of the complete psychological works of the Sigmund Freud: Vol. XIX (1923–1925): The ego and the id and other works*. Hogarth Press.

Geller, J. D., & Gould, E. (1996). A contemporary psychoanalytic perspective: Rogers' brief psychotherapy with Mary Jane Tilden. In B. A. Farber, D. C. Brink, & P. M. Raskin (Eds.), *The psychotherapy of Carl Rogers: Cases and commentary* (pp. 211–230). Guilford Press.

Geller, S. (2020). Cultivating online therapeutic presence: Strengthening therapeutic relationships in teletherapy sessions. *Counselling Psychology Quarterly*. Advance online publication. https://doi.org/10.1080/09515070.2020.1787348

Geller, S. M. (2013). Therapeutic presence: An essential way of being. In M. Cooper, P. F. Schmid, M. O'Hara, & A. C. Bohart (Eds.), *The handbook of person-centred psychotherapy and counselling* (2nd ed., pp. 209–222). Palgrave Macmillan/Springer Nature. https://doi.org/10.1007/978-1-137-32900-4_14

Geller, S. M., & Greenberg, L. S. (2012). *Therapeutic presence: A mindful approach to effective therapy*. American Psychological Association. https://doi.org/10.1037/13485-000

Geller, S. M., Greenberg, L. S., & Watson, J. C. (2010). Therapist and client perceptions of therapeutic presence: The development of a measure. *Journal of Psychotherapy Research, 20*(5), 599–610. https://doi.org/10.1080/10503307.2010.495957

Gelso, C. J. (2011). *The real relationship in psychotherapy: The hidden foundation of change*. American Psychological Association. https://doi.org/10.1037/12349-000

Gelso, C. J. (2019). *The therapeutic relationship in psychotherapeutic practice: An integrative perspective*. Routledge.

Gelso, C. J., Kivlighan, D. M., & Markin, R. D. (2019). The real relationship. In J. C. Norcross & M. J. Lambert (Eds.), *Psychotherapy relationships that work: Vol. 1. Evidence-based therapist contributions* (3rd ed., pp. 351–378). Oxford University Press. https://doi.org/10.1093/med-psych/9780190843953.003.0010

Gendlin, E. T. (1970). A short summary and some long predictions. In J. T. Hart & T. M. Tomlinson (Eds.), *New directions in client-centered therapy* (pp. 544–562). Houghton Mifflin.

Gendlin, E. T. (1978). *Focusing*. Everest House.

Gendlin, E. T. (1996). *Focusing-oriented psychotherapy: A manual of the experiential method*. Guilford Press.

Germain, V., Marchand, A., Bouchard, S., Guay, S., & Drouin, M. S. (2010). Assessment of the therapeutic alliance in face-to-face or videoconference treatment for posttraumatic stress disorder. *Cyberpsychology, Behavior, and Social Networking, 13*(1), 29–35. https://doi.org/10.1089/cyber.2009.0139

Goldfried, M. R., & Davila, J. (2005). The role of relationship and technique in therapeutic change. *Psychotherapy: Theory, Research, Practice, Training, 42*(4), 421–430. https://doi.org/10.1037/0033-3204.42.4.421

Goldstein, F., & Glueck, D. (2016). Developing rapport and therapeutic alliance during telemental health sessions with children and adolescents. *Journal of Child and Adolescent Psychopharmacology, 26*(3), 204–211. https://doi.org/10.1089/cap.2015.0022

Gottlieb, L. (2019). *Maybe you should talk to someone: A therapist, her therapist, and our lives revealed*. Houghton Mifflin.

Greenberg, L. S. (2002). Integrating an emotion-focused approach to treatment into psychotherapy integration. *Journal of Psychotherapy Integration, 12*(2), 154–189. https://doi.org/10.1037/1053-0479.12.2.154

Greenberg, L. S. (2016). *Emotion-focused therapy*. American Psychological Association.

Guntrip, H. (1996). My experience of analysis with Fairbairn and Winnicott (How complete a result does psychoanalytic therapy achieve?). *The International Journal of Psychoanalysis, 77*(4), 739–754. https://icpla.edu/wp-content/uploads/2012/10/Guntrip-H.-My-Experience-of-Analysis-with-Fairbairn-and-Winnicott-Int.J.Psychoa.-vol.77-p.739-1996.pdf

Gurman, A. S. (1977). The patient's perception of the therapeutic relationship. In A. S. Gurman & A. M. Razin (Eds.), *Effective psychotherapy: A handbook of research* (pp. 503–543). Pergamon.

Hall, J., & Leary, M. (2020, September 17). The U.S. has an empathy deficit. *Scientific American*. https://www.scientificamerican.com/article/the-us-has-an-empathy-deficit/

Heine, S. J., Lehman, D. R., Markus, H. R., & Kitayama, S. (1999). Is there a universal need for positive self-regard? *Psychological Review, 106*(4), 766–794. https://doi.org/10.1037/0033-295X.106.4.766

Hendricks, M. (2001). An experiential version of unconditional positive regard. In J. D. Bozarth & P. Wilkins (Eds.), *Rogers' therapeutic conditions: Evolution, theory and practice: Vol. 3. Unconditional positive regard* (pp. 126–144). PCCS Books.

Henretty, J. R., & Levitt, H. M. (2010). The role of therapist self-disclosure in psychotherapy: A qualitative review. *Clinical Psychology Review, 30*(1), 63–77. https://doi.org/10.1016/j.cpr.2009.09.004

Henriques, G. (2012, June 23). Relational value: A core human need. *Psychology Today.* https://www.psychologytoday.com/us/blog/theory-knowledge/201206/relational-value

Hill, C. E. (2020). *Helping skills: Facilitating exploration, insight, and action* (5th ed.). American Psychological Association. https://doi.org/10.1037/0000147-000

Hill, C. E., Knox, S., Thompson, B. J., Williams, E. N., Hess, S. A., & Ladany, N. (2005). Consensual qualitative research: An update. *Journal of Counseling Psychology, 52*(2), 196–205.

Hill, C. E., Thompson, B. J., Cogar, M. C., & Denman, D. W. (1993). Beneath the surface of long-term therapy: Therapist and client report of their own and each other's covert processes. *Journal of Counseling Psychology, 40*(3), 278–287. https://doi.org/10.1037/0022-0167.40.3.278

Hollenbaugh, E. E., & Everett, M. K. (2013). The effects of anonymity on self-disclosure in blogs: An application of the online disinhibition effect. *Journal of Computer-Mediated Communication, 18*(3), 283–302. https://doi.org/10.1111/jcc4.12008

Iberg, J. R. (2001). Unconditional positive regard: Constituent activities. In J. D. Bozarth & P. Wilkins (Eds.), *Rogers' therapeutic conditions: Evolution, theory and practice: Vol. 3. Unconditional positive regard* (pp. 109–125). PCCS Books.

Jackson, D., Farber, B. A., & Mandavia, A. (2022). The nature, motives, and perceived consequences of therapist dishonesty. *Psychotherapy Research, 32*(3), 372–388. https://doi.org/10.1080/10503307.2021.1933241

Jaison, B. (2008). Getting the most from the therapy hour: Integrating experiential and brief therapy. In K. Tudor (Ed.), *Brief person-centred therapies* (pp. 47–63). SAGE. https://doi.org/10.4135/9781446221297.n4

James, W. (1981). *The principles of psychology*. Harvard University Press. (Original work published 1890)

Jefferson Airplane. (1969). Wooden ships [Song]. On *Volunteers*. RCA.

Johnson, S. M. (2009). Attachment theory and emotionally focused therapy for individuals and couples: Perfect partners. In J. H. Obegi & E. Berant (Eds.), *Attachment theory and research in clinical work with adults* (pp. 410–433). Guilford Press.

Johnson, S. M. (2019). *Attachment theory in practice: Emotionally focused therapy (EFT) with individuals, couples, and families*. Guilford Press.

Josefowitz, N., & Myran, D. (2005). Towards a person-centred cognitive behaviour therapy. *Counselling Psychology Quarterly, 18*(4), 329–336. https://doi.org/10.1080/09515070500473600

Junod, T. (2019, November 18). My friend Mister Rogers. *The Atlantic.* https://www.theatlantic.com/magazine/archive/2019/12/what-would-mister-rogers-do/600772/

Kalman, Y. M., & Rafaeli, S. (2011). Online pauses and silence: Chronemic expectancy violations in written computer-mediated communication. *Communication Research, 38*(1), 54–69. https://doi.org/10.1177/0093650210378229

Kariagina, T. D. (2017). Where empathy in psychotherapy originated: C. Rogers, his psychoanalytic predecessors and followers. *Journal of Russian & East European Psychology, 54*(6), 498–526. https://doi.org/10.1080/10610405.2017.1448183

Kayany, J. M., Wotring, C. E., & Forrest, E. J. (1996). Relational control and interactive media choice in technology-mediated communication situations. *Human Communication Research, 22*(3), 399–421. https://doi.org/10.1111/j.1468-2958.1996.tb00373.x

Kensit, D. A. (2000). Rogerian theory: A critique of the effectiveness of pure client-centred therapy. *Counselling Psychology Quarterly, 13*(4), 345–351. https://doi.org/10.1080/713658499

Kernberg, O. F. (1976). Technical considerations in the treatment of borderline personality organization. *Journal of the American Psychoanalytic Association, 24*(4), 795–829. https://doi.org/10.1177/000306517602400403

Kettler, Sara. (2020, June 24). *Fred Rogers took a stand against racial inequality when he invited a Black character to join him in a pool.* Biography. https://www.biography.com/news/mister-rogers-officer-clemmons-pool

King, M. (2018). *The good neighbor: The life and work of Fred Rogers.* Abrams Press.

Kirschenbaum, H. (1979). *On becoming Carl Rogers.* Delacorte.

Kirschenbaum, H. (2007). *The life and work of Carl Rogers.* PCCS Books.

Kirschenbaum, H., & Henderson, V. L. (Eds.). (1989). *Carl Rogers: Dialogues: Conversations with Martin Buber, Paul Tillich, B. F. Skinner, Gregory Bateson, Michael Polanyi, Rollo May, and others.* Houghton Mifflin.

Klein, E. (2021, February 19). What it means to be kind in a cruel world. *The New York Times.* https://www.nytimes.com/2021/02/19/opinion/ezra-klein-podcast-george-saunders.html

Knausgaard, K. O. (2013). *My struggle: Book 1* (D. Bartlett, Trans.). Farrar, Straus and Giroux. (Original work published 2009)

Knox, S., & Hill, C. E. (2003). Therapist self-disclosure: Research-based suggestions for practitioners. *Journal of Clinical Psychology, 59*(5), 529–539. https://doi.org/10.1002/jclp.10157

Kohut, H. (1959). Introspection, empathy, and psychoanalysis: An examination of the relationship between mode of observation and theory. *Journal of the American Psychoanalytic Association, 7*(3), 459–483. https://doi.org/10.1177/000306515900700304

Kohut, H. (1971). *The analysis of the self: A systematic approach to the psychoanalytic treatment of narcissistic personality disorders.* International Universities Press.

Kohut, H. (1977). *The restoration of the self.* International Universities Press.

Kolden, G. G., Wang, C.-C., Austin, S. B., Chang, Y., & Klein, M. H. (2019). Congruence/genuineness. In J. C. Norcross & M. J. Lambert (Eds.), *Psychotherapy relationships that work: Vol. 1. Evidence-based therapist contributions* (3rd ed., pp. 323–350). Oxford University Press. https://doi.org/10.1093/med-psych/9780190843953.003.0009

Kramer, R. (1995). The birth of client-centered therapy: Carl Rogers, Otto Rank, and "the beyond." *Journal of Humanistic Psychology, 35*(4), 54–110. https://doi.org/10.1177/00221678950354005

Lambert, M. J. (2003). *Bergin and Garfield's handbook of psychotherapy and behavior change* (5th ed.). John Wiley.

Lambert, M. J. (2013). The efficacy and effectiveness of psychotherapy. In M. J. Lambert (Ed.), *Bergin and Garfield's handbook of psychotherapy and behavior change* (6th ed., pp. 139–193). Wiley.

Lane, J. S., Farber, B. A., & Geller, J. D. (2001, June 20–24). *What therapists do and don't disclose to their patients* [Paper presentation]. Society for Psychotherapy Research 32nd Annual Meeting, Montevideo, Uruguay.

Leary, M. R., & Allen, A. B. (2011). Belonging motivation: Establishing, maintaining, and repairing relational value. In D. Dunning (Ed.), *Frontiers of social psychology. Social motivation* (pp. 37–55). Psychology Press.

Lees, J. (2005). A history of psychoanalytic research. *Psychodynamic Practice, 11*(2), 117–131. https://doi.org/10.1080/14753630500108042

LeFebvre, L. E., Allen, M., Rasner, R. D., Garstad, S., Wilms, A., & Parrish, C. (2019). Ghosting in emerging adults' romantic relationships: The digital dissolution disappearance strategy. *Imagination, Cognition and Personality, 39*(2), 125–150. https://doi.org/10.1177/0276236618820519

Leiper, R., & Casares, P. (2000). An investigation of the attachment organization of clinical psychologists and its relationship to clinical practice. *The British Journal of Medical Psychology, 73*(4), 449–464. https://doi.org/10.1348/000711200160651

Lemoire, S. J., & Chen, C. P. (2005). Applying person-centered counseling to sexual minority adolescents. *Journal of Counseling & Development, 83*(2), 146–154. https://doi.org/10.1002/j.1556-6678.2005.tb00591.x

Levant, R. F., & Shlien, J. M. (Eds.). (1984). *Client-centered therapy and the person-centered approach: New directions in theory, research, and practice.* Praeger.

Lietaer, G. (1984). Unconditional positive regard: A controversial basic attitude in client-centered therapy. In R. F. Levant & J. M. Shlien (Eds.), *Client-centered therapy and the person-centered approach: New directions in theory, research, and practice* (pp. 41–58). Praeger.

Lietaer, G. (2001). Unconditional acceptance and positive regard. In J. D. Bozarth & P. Wilkins (Eds.), *Rogers' therapeutic conditions: Evolution, theory and practice: Vol. 3. Unconditional positive regard* (pp. 88–108). PCCS Books.

Lietaer, G., & Gundrum, M. (2018). His master's voice: Carl Rogers' verbal response modes in therapy and demonstration sessions throughout his career. A quantitative analysis and some qualitative-clinical comments. *Person-Centered & Experiential Psychotherapies, 17*(4), 275–333. https://doi.org/10.1080/14779757.2018.1544091

Linehan, M. M. (1993). *Cognitive-behavioral treatment of borderline personality disorder*. Guilford Press.

Linehan, M. M. (2006). *Treating borderline personality disorder: The dialectical approach* [Film; educational DVD]. Guilford Press.

MacDonald, J., & Morley, I. (2001). Shame and non-disclosure: A study of the emotional isolation of people referred for psychotherapy. *British Journal of Medical Psychology, 74*(1), 1–21. https://doi.org/10.1348/000711201160731

MacKinnon, D. W., & Dukes, W. F. (1962). Repression. In L. E. Postman (Ed.), *Psychology in the making* (pp. 662–744). Knopf.

Macran, S., & Shapiro, D. A. (1998). The role of personal therapy for therapists: A review. *The British Journal of Medical Psychology, 71*(1), 13–25. https://doi.org/10.1111/j.2044-8341.1998.tb01364.x

Marmarosh, C. L., & Kivlighan, D. M., Jr. (2012). Relationships among client and counselor agreement about the working alliance, session evaluations, and change in client symptoms using response surface analysis. *Journal of Counseling Psychology, 59*(3), 352–367. https://doi.org/10.1037/a0028907

May, R. (1982). The problem of evil: An open letter to Carl Rogers. *Journal of Humanistic Psychology, 22*(3), 10–21. https://doi.org/10.1177/0022167882223003

McLuhan, M., & Fiore, Q. (1967). *The medium is the massage: An inventory of effects*. Bantam Books.

McMullen, L., & Ort, D. (2021, June 23–26). *Therapist ghosting* [Paper presentation]. Society for Psychotherapy Research 52nd Annual International Meeting, Heidelberg, Germany.

McWilliams, N. (2004). *Psychoanalytic psychotherapy: A practitioner's guide*. Guilford Press.

Mearns, D. (1994). *Developing person-centred counselling*. SAGE.

Mearns, D., & Cooper, M. (2005). *Working at relational depth in counseling and psychotherapy*. SAGE.

Mearns, D., & Thorne, B. (2000). *Person-centred therapy today: New frontiers in theory and practice*. SAGE.

Mearns, D., & Thorne, B. (2007). *Person-centred counselling in action* (3rd ed.). SAGE.

Miller, A. (1997). *The drama of the gifted child: The search for the true self* (3rd ed.). Basic Books. (Original work published 1981 as *Prisoners of childhood: The drama of the gifted child and the search for the true self*)

Miller, W. R. (2000). Rediscovering fire: Small interventions, large effects. *Psychology of Addictive Behaviors, 14*(1), 6–18. https://doi.org/10.1037/0893-164X.14.1.6

Mitchell, K. M., Bozarth, J. D., & Krauft, C. C. (1977). A reappraisal of the therapeutic effectiveness of accurate empathy, nonpossessive warmth and genuineness. In A. S. Gurman & A. M. Razin (Eds.), *Effective psychotherapy* (pp. 482–502). Pergamon.

Mitchell, S. A. (2000). *Relationality: From attachment to intersubjectivity*. Analytic Press.

Mitchell, S. A., & Black, M. J. (1995). *Freud and beyond.* Basic Books.

Modell, A. H. (1976). "The Holding Environment" and the therapeutic action of psychoanalysis. *Journal of the American Psychoanalytic Association, 24*(2), 285–307. https://doi.org/10.1177/000306517602400202

Momigliano, L. N. (1987). A spell in Vienna—But was Freud a Freudian? *The International Review of Psycho-Analysis, 14,* 373–388.

Morgan, P. (Writer), & Jarrold, J. (Director). (2016, November 4). Act of God (Season 1, Episode 4) [TV series episode]. In P. Morgan (Executive Producer), *The crown.* Left Bank Pictures; Sony Pictures Television.

Murphy, D., Joseph, S., Demetriou, E., & Karimi-Mofrad, P. (2020). Unconditional positive self-regard, intrinsic aspirations, and authenticity: Pathways to psychological well-being. *Journal of Humanistic Psychology, 60*(2), 258–279. https://doi.org/10.1177/0022167816688314

Ng, C. (2017). *Little fires everywhere.* Penguin.

Nitzburg, G. C., & Farber, B. A. (2019). Patterns of utilization and a case illustration of an interactive text-based psychotherapy delivery system. *Journal of Clinical Psychology, 75*(2), 247–259. https://doi.org/10.1002/jclp.22718

Norcross, J. C. (Ed.). (2002). *Psychotherapy relationships that work: Therapist contributions and responsiveness to patients.* Oxford University Press.

Norcross, J. C. (Ed.). (2011). *Psychotherapy relationships that work: Evidence-based responsiveness* (2nd ed.). Oxford University Press. https://doi.org/10.1093/acprof:oso/9780199737208.001.0001

Norcross, J. C., & Lambert, M. J. (2018). Psychotherapy relationships that work III. *Psychotherapy, 55*(4), 303–315. https://doi.org/10.1037/pst0000193

Norcross, J. C., & Lambert, M. J. (Eds.). (2019). *Psychotherapy relationships that work: Vol. 1. Evidence-based therapist contributions* (3rd ed.). Oxford University Press.

Norcross, J. C., & Wampold, B. E. (Eds.). (2019). *Psychotherapy relationships that work: Vol. 2. Evidence-based therapist responsiveness* (3rd ed.). Oxford University Press.

Openshaw, D. K., Morrow, J., Law, D., Moen, D., Johnson, C., & Talley, S. (2012). Examining the satisfaction of women residing in rural Utah who received therapy for depression through teletherapy. *Rural Mental Health, 36*(2), 38–45. https://doi.org/10.1037/h0095814

Orange, T. (2018). *There there: A novel.* Vintage Books.

Orlinsky, D. E., Grawe, K., & Parks, B. K. (1994). Process and outcome in psychotherapy: Noch einmal. In A. E. Bergin & S. L. Garfield (Eds.), *Handbook of psychotherapy and behavior change* (4th ed., pp. 270–376). John Wiley & Sons.

Orlinsky, D. E., & Howard, K. I. (1978). The relation of process to outcome in psychotherapy. In A. E. Bergin & S. L. Garfield (Eds.), *Handbook of psychotherapy and behavior change: An empirical analysis* (2nd ed., pp. 283–330). John Wiley & Sons.

Orlinsky, D. E., & Howard, K. I. (1986). Process and outcome in psychotherapy. In S. L. Garfield & A. E. Bergin (Eds.), *Handbook of psychological behavior and change* (3rd ed., pp. 311–381). John Wiley & Sons.

Ort, D., & Farber, B. A. (2021, June 23–26). *Teletherapy during COVID-19* [Paper presentation]. Society for Psychotherapy Research 52nd Annual International Meeting, Heidelberg, Germany.

O'Sullivan, P. B., Hunt, S. K., & Lippert, L. R. (2004). Mediated immediacy: A language of affiliation in a technological age. *Journal of Language and Social Psychology, 23*(4), 464–490. https://doi.org/10.1177/0261927X04269588

Palmer, E. L., & Carr, K. (1991). Dr. Rogers, meet Mr. Rogers: The theoretical and clinical similarities between Carl and Fred Rogers. *Social Behavior and Personality, 19*(1), 39–44. https://doi.org/10.2224/sbp.1991.19.1.39

Pancani, L., Marinucci, M., Aureli, N., & Riva, P. (2021). Forced social isolation and mental health: A study on 1,006 Italians under COVID-19 lockdown. *Frontiers in Psychology.* https://doi.org/10.3389/fpsyg.2021.663799

Panichelli, C., Albert, A., Donneau, A.-F., D'Amore, S., Triffaux, J.-M., & Ansseau, M. (2018). Humor associated with positive outcomes in individual psychotherapy. *American Journal of Psychotherapy, 71*(3), 95–103. https://doi.org/10.1176/appi.psychotherapy.20180021

Parloff, M. B., Waskow, I. E., & Wolfe, B. E. (1978). Research on therapist variables in relation to process and outcome. In S. L. Garfield & A. E. Bergin (Eds.), *Handbook of psychotherapy and behavior change: An empirical analysis* (2nd ed., pp. 233–282). John Wiley & Sons.

Patterson, T. G., & Joseph, S. (2006). Development of a self-report measure of unconditional positive self-regard. *Psychology and Psychotherapy: Theory, Research and Practice, 79*(4), 557–570. https://doi.org/10.1348/147608305X89414

Paul, G. L. (1967). Strategy of outcome research in psychotherapy. *Journal of Consulting Psychology, 31*(2), 109–118. https://doi.org/10.1037/h0024436

Pedersen, P. (1996). The importance of both similarities and differences in multicultural counseling: Reaction to C. H. Patterson. *Journal of Counseling and Development, 74*(3), 236–237.

Polack, E. (2018, May 1). *New Cigna study reveals loneliness at epidemic levels in America.* https://www.cigna.com/about-us/newsroom/news-and-views/press-releases/2018/new-cigna-study-reveals-loneliness-at-epidemic-levels-in-america

Pope, K. S., Tabachnick, B. G., & Keith-Spiegel, P. (1987). Ethics of practice: The beliefs and behaviors of psychologists as therapists. *American Psychologist, 42*(11), 993–1006. https://doi.org/10.1037/0003-066X.42.11.993

Pounds, G., Hunt, D., & Koteyko, N. (2018). Expression of empathy in a Facebook-based diabetes support group. *Discourse, Context & Media, 25*, 34–43. https://doi.org/10.1016/j.dcm.2018.01.008

Prunetti, E., Framba, R., Barone, L., Fiore, D., Sera, F., & Liotti, G. (2008). Attachment disorganization and borderline patients' metacognitive responses to therapists' expressed understanding of their states of mind: A pilot study. *Psychotherapy Research, 18*(1), 28–36. https://doi.org/10.1080/10503300701320645

Rank, O. (1978). *Will therapy: An analysis of the therapeutic process in terms of relationship* (J. Taft, Trans.). W. W. Norton. (Original work published 1936)

Raskin, N. J. (1948). The development of nondirective therapy. *Journal of Consulting Psychology, 12*(2), 92–110. https://doi.org/10.1037/h0058003

Raskin, N. J. (1987). From spyglass to kaleidoscope [Review of *Client-centered therapy and the person-centered approach: New directions in theory, research, and practice* by R. F. Levant & J. M. Shlien (Eds.)]. *Contemporary Psychology, 32*(5), 460–461. https://doi.org/10.1037/027145

Redford, R. (1980). *Ordinary people* [Film]. Wildwood Enterprises.

Rogers, C. R. (1942). *Counseling and psychotherapy: Newer concepts in practice.* Houghton Mifflin Company.

Rogers, C. R. (1951). *Client-centered therapy: Its current practice, implications, and theory.* Houghton Mifflin.

Rogers, C. R. (1957). The necessary and sufficient conditions of therapeutic personality change. *Journal of Consulting Psychology, 21*(2), 95–103. https://doi.org/10.1037/h0045357

Rogers, C. R. (1959). A theory of therapy, personality, and interpersonal relationships, as developed in the client-centered framework. In S. Koch (Ed.), *Psychology: A study of a science. Study 1: Formulations of the person and the social context* (Vol. 3, pp. 184–256). McGraw Hill.

Rogers, C. R. (1961). *On becoming a person: A therapist's view of psychotherapy.* Houghton Mifflin.

Rogers, C. R. (1967). A silent young man. In C. R. Rogers, E. T. Gendlin, D. J. Kiesler, & C. B. Truax (Eds.), *The therapeutic relationship and its impact: A study of psychotherapy with schizophrenics* (pp. 401–416). University of Wisconsin Press.

Rogers, C. R. (1970). *Carl Rogers on encounter groups.* Harper & Row.

Rogers, C. R. (1980). *A way of being.* Houghton Mifflin.

Rogers, C. R. (1986). Reflection of feelings. *Person-Centered Review, 1*(4), 375–377.

Rogers, C. R. (1987). Rogers, Kohut, and Erickson: A personal perspective on some similarities and differences. In J. K. Zeig (Ed.), *The evolution of psychotherapy* (pp. 179–187). Routledge.

Rogers, C. R. (1989). *The Carl Rogers reader* (H. Kirschenbaum & V. L. Henderson, Eds.). Houghton Mifflin.

Rogers, C. R., & Dymond, R. F. (1954). *Psychotherapy and personality change.* Amsterdam University Press.

Rogers, C. R., Gendlin, E. T., Kiesler, D. J., & Truax, C. B. (Eds.). (1967). *The therapeutic relationship and its impact: A study of psychotherapy with schizophrenics.* University of Wisconsin Press.

Rogers, C. R., & Hart, J. (1970). Looking back and ahead: A conversation with Carl Rogers. In J. T. Hart & T. M. Tomlinson (Eds.), *New directions in client-centered therapy* (pp. 502–534). Houghton Mifflin.

Rogers, C. R., & Russell, D. E. (2002). *Carl Rogers: The quiet revolutionary: An oral history.* Penmarin Books.

Rogers, F. (2019). *A beautiful day in the neighborhood: Neighborly words of wisdom from Mister Rogers.* Penguin Books.

Roos, J., & Werbart, A. (2013). Therapist and relationship factors influencing dropout from individual psychotherapy: A literature review. *Psychotherapy Research, 23*(4), 394–418. https://doi.org/10.1080/10503307.2013.775528

Roth, G., Assor, A., Niemiec, C. P., Ryan, R. M., & Deci, E. L. (2009). The emotional and academic consequences of parental conditional regard: Comparing conditional positive regard, conditional negative regard, and autonomy support as parenting practices. *Developmental Psychology, 45*(4), 1119–1142. https://doi.org/10.1037/a0015272

Safran, J. D., & Muran, J. C. (2000). *Negotiating the therapeutic alliance: A relational treatment guide.* Guilford Press.

Sanford, R. (2001). Unconditional positive regard: A misunderstood way of being. In J. D. Bozarth & P. Wilkins (Eds.), *Rogers' therapeutic conditions: Evolution, theory and practice: Vol. 3. Unconditional positive regard* (pp. 65–75). PCCS Books.

Schmid, P. F. (2004). Back to the client: A phenomenological approach to the process of understanding and diagnosis. *Person-Centered & Experiential Psychotherapies, 3*(1), 36–51.

Schneider, K. (2013). *The polarized mind: Why it's killing us and what we can do about it.* University Professors Press.

Schneider, K. (2015). Presence: The core contextual factor of effective psychotherapy. *Existential Analysis, 26*(2), 304–312.

Schwartz-Mette, R. A., & Shen-Miller, D. S. (2018). Ships in the rising sea? Changes over time in psychologists' ethical beliefs and behaviors. *Ethics & Behavior, 28*(3), 176–198. https://doi.org/10.1080/10508422.2017.1308253

Shakespeare, W. (2003). *Macbeth.* Simon & Schuster. (Original work published 1623)

Shostrom, E. (Director). (1965). *Three approaches to psychotherapy* [Film]. Psychological Films.

Simon, P. (1983). Hearts and bones [Song]. On *Hearts and Bones.* Warner Brothers.

Simpson, S. G., & Reid, C. L. (2014). Therapeutic alliance in videoconferencing psychotherapy: A review. *The Australian Journal of Rural Health, 22*(6), 280–299. https://doi.org/10.1111/ajr.12149

Slatcher, R. B., Vazire, S., & Pennebaker, J. W. (2008). Am "I" more important than "we"? Couples' word use in instant messages. *Personal Relationships, 15*(4), 407–424. https://doi.org/10.1111/j.1475-6811.2008.00207.x

Smith, M. L., & Glass, G. V. (1980). Meta-analysis of research on class size and its relationship to attitudes and instruction. *American Educational Research Journal, 17*(4), 419–433. https://doi.org/10.3102/00028312017004419

Snyder, W. (1947). *Casebook of non-directive counseling.* Houghton Mifflin.

Standal, S. W. (1954). *The need for positive regard: A contribution to client-centered theory* [Unpublished doctoral dissertation]. The University of Chicago.

Staples, F. R., Sloane, R. B., Whipple, K., Cristol, A. H., & Yorkston, N. J. (1975). Differences between behavior therapists and psychotherapists. *Archives of General Psychiatry, 32*(12), 1517–1522. https://doi.org/10.1001/archpsyc.1975.01760300055003

Stern, D. N. (1985). *The interpersonal world of the infant: A view from psychoanalysis and developmental psychology.* Basic Books.

Stiles, W. B., Honos-Webb, L., & Surko, M. (1998). Responsiveness in psychotherapy. *Clinical Psychology: Science and Practice, 5*(4), 439–458. https://doi.org/10.1111/j.1468-2850.1998.tb00166.x

Stolorow, R. D. (1976). Psychoanalytic reflections on client-centered therapy in the light of modern conceptions of narcissism. *Psychotherapy: Theory, Research & Practice, 13*(1), 26–29. https://doi.org/10.1037/h0086479

Storr, A. (2001). *Freud: A very short introduction.* Oxford University Press. https://doi.org/10.1093/actrade/9780192854551.001.0001

Sue, D. W., Sue, D., Neville, H. A., & Smith, L. (2019). *Counseling the culturally diverse: Theory and practice.* John Wiley & Sons.

Suh, C. S., O'Malley, S. S., Strupp, H. H., & Johnson, M. E. (1989). The Vanderbilt Psychotherapy Process Scale (VPPS). *Journal of Cognitive Psychotherapy, 3*(2), 123–154. https://doi.org/10.1891/0889-8391.3.2.123

Suler, J. (2004). The online disinhibition effect. *CyberPsychology & Behavior, 7*(3), 321–326. https://doi.org/10.1089/1094931041291295

Suzuki, J. Y. (2018). *A qualitative investigation of psychotherapy clients' perceptions of positive regard* (Publication No. 10840096) [Doctoral dissertation, Columbia University]. ProQuest Dissertations and Theses Global.

Suzuki, J. Y., & Farber, B. A. (2016). Toward greater specificity of the concept of positive regard. *Person-Centered & Experiential Psychotherapies, 15*(4), 263–284. https://doi.org/10.1080/14779757.2016.1204941

Suzuki, J. Y., Mandavia, A., & Farber, B. A. (2019). Clients' perceptions of positive regard across four therapeutic orientations. *Journal of Psychotherapy Integration.* Advance online publication. https://doi.org/10.1037/int0000186

Timulák, L., & Lietaer, G. (2001). Moments of empowerment: A qualitative analysis of positively experienced episodes in brief person-centred counselling. *Counselling & Psychotherapy Research, 1*(1), 62–73. https://doi.org/10.1080/14733140112331385268

Tobin, S. A. (1991). A comparison of psychoanalytic self psychology and Carl Rogers's person-centered therapy. *Journal of Humanistic Psychology, 31*(1), 9–33. https://doi.org/10.1177/0022167891311002

Truax, C. B. (1966). Reinforcement and nonreinforcement in Rogerian psychotherapy. *Journal of Abnormal Psychology, 71*(1), 1–9. https://doi.org/10.1037/h0022912

Truax, C. B., & Carkhuff, R. R. (1967). *Toward effective counseling and psychotherapy: Training and practice.* Aldine Publishing Company.

Truax, C. B., & Mitchell, K. M. (1971). Research on certain therapist interpersonal skills in relation to process and outcome. In A. E. Bergin & S. L. Garfield (Eds.), *Handbook of psychotherapy and behavior change* (pp. 299–344). John Wiley & Sons.

Truax, C. B., Wargo, D. G., Frank, J. D., Imber, S. D., Battle, C. C., Hoehn-Saric, R., Nash, E. H., & Stone, A. R. (1966). Therapist empathy, genuineness, and warmth and patient therapeutic outcome. *Journal of Consulting Psychology, 30*(5), 395–401. https://doi.org/10.1037/h0023827

Velasquez, P. A. E., & Montiel, C. J. (2018). Reapproaching Rogers: A discursive examination of client-centered therapy. *Person-Centered & Experiential Psychotherapies, 17*(3), 253–269. https://doi.org/10.1080/14779757.2018.1527243

Wachtel, P. L. (2007). Carl Rogers and the larger context of therapeutic thought. *Psychotherapy: Theory, Research, & Practice, 44*(3), 279–284. https://doi.org/10.1037/0033-3204.44.3.279

Wachtel, P. L. (2008). *Relational theory and the practice of psychotherapy*. Guilford Press.

Wachtel, P. L. (2011). *Therapeutic communication: Knowing what to say when* (2nd ed.). Guilford Press.

Wachtel, P. L. (2014). An integrative relational point of view. *Psychotherapy: Theory, Research, & Practice, 51*(3), 342–349. https://doi.org/10.1037/a0037219

Walfish, S., McAlister, B., O'Donnell, P., & Lambert, M. J. (2012). An investigation of self-assessment bias in mental health providers. *Psychological Reports, 110*(2), 639–644. https://doi.org/10.2466/02.07.17.PR0.110.2.639-644

Walther, J. B., & Tidwell, L. C. (1995). Nonverbal cues in computer-mediated communication, and the effect of chronemics on relational communication. *Journal of Organizational Computing, 5*(4), 355–378. https://doi.org/10.1080/10919399509540258

Wampold, B. E., & Imel, Z. E. (2015). *The great psychotherapy debate: The evidence for what makes psychotherapy work* (2nd ed.). Routledge. https://doi.org/10.4324/9780203582015

Watkins, G. (1987). *Dickens in search of himself: Recurrent themes and characters in the work of Charles Dickens*. Palgrave Macmillan. https://doi.org/10.1007/978-1-349-08550-7

Watson, J. C. (1999). *Measure of expressed empathy*. Department of Adult Education, Community Development, and Counseling Psychology, OISE, University of Toronto.

Watson, J. C., & Geller, S. M. (2005). The relation among the relationship conditions, working alliance, and outcome in both process–experiential and cognitive–behavioral psychotherapies. *Psychotherapy Research, 15*(1-2), 25–33. https://doi.org/10.1080/10503300512331327010

Watson, J. C., & Greenberg, L. S. (2009). Empathic resonance: A neuroscience perspective. In J. Decety & W. Ickes (Eds.), *The social neuroscience of empathy* (pp. 125–137). MIT Press. https://doi.org/10.7551/mitpress/9780262012973.003.0011

Watson, J. C., McMullen, E. J., Rodrigues, A., & Prosser, M. C. (2020). Examining the role of therapists' empathy and clients' attachment styles on changes in clients' affect regulation and outcome in the treatment of depression. *Psychotherapy Research, 30*(6), 693–705. https://doi.org/10.1080/10503307.2019.1658912

Watson, J. C., Steckley, P. L., & McMullen, E. J. (2014). The role of empathy in promoting change. *Psychotherapy Research, 24*(3), 286–298. https://doi.org/10.1080/10503307.2013.802823

Weber Shandwick. (2018, June 13). *Civility in America 2018: Civility at work and in our public squares.* https://www.webershandwick.com/news/civility-in-america-2018-civility-at-work-and-in-our-public-squares/

Wenzel, A. (2016). *Cognitive behavioral therapy over time* [Film; educational DVD]. American Psychological Association.

Westover, T. (2018). *Educated: A memoir.* Random House.

Whiteley, J. M. (Producer). (1977). *Carl Rogers counsels an individual on anger and hurt* [Film]. American Personnel and Guidance Association.

Whiteley, J. M. (Producer). (1980). *Sylvia: The struggle for self acceptance* [Film]. American Association for Counseling and Development.

Whitman, W. (1855). *Leaves of grass: The original 1855 edition (chump change edition).* Ross Bolton.

Wilkins, P. (2001). Unconditional positive regard reconsidered. In J. D. Bozarth & P. Wilkins (Eds.), *Rogers' therapeutic conditions: Evolution, theory and practice: Vol. 3. Unconditional positive regard* (pp. 35–48). PCCS Books. (Reprinted from "Unconditional positive regard reconsidered," 2000, *British Journal of Guidance & Counselling, 28*[1], 23–36, https://doi.org/10.1080/030698800109592)

Wilkins, P. (2010). *Person-centred therapy: 100 key points.* Routledge.

Williams, T. (1947). *A streetcar named Desire.* Signet.

Winnicott, D. W. (1955). Group influences and the maladjusted child: The school aspect. In L. Caldwell & H. Taylor Robinson (Eds.) (2017), *The collected works of D. W. Winnicott: Vol. 5. 1955–1959* (pp. 19–114). Oxford University Press.

Winnicott, D. W. (1960). The theory of the parent–infant relationship. *The International Journal of Psycho-Analysis, 41,* 585–595.

Winnicott, D. W. (1965). *The maturational processes and the facilitating environment.* Karnac Books.

Winnicott, D. W. (1969). The use of an object. *The International Journal of Psycho-Analysis, 50*(4), 711–716.

Winnicott, D. W. (1990). *Home is where we start from.* W. W. Norton.

Wise, T. L. (2012). *Waking up: Climbing through the darkness.* Missing Peace.

Yalom, I. D. (1980). *Existential psychotherapy.* Basic Books.

Yalom, I. D. (1992). *When Nietzsche wept.* Basic Books.

Yalom, I. D. (1995). *The theory and practice of group psychotherapy* (4th ed.). Basic Books.

Yalom, I. D. (2002). *The gift of therapy: An open letter to a new generation of therapists and their patients.* HarperCollins.

Yalom, I. D. (2005). *The Schopenhauer cure: A novel.* Harper.

Yalom, I. D. (2012). *Love's executioner and other tales of psychotherapy.* Basic Books.

Yalom, I. D. (2020). *Momma and the meaning of life: Tales of psychotherapy.* Harper Perennial.

Yassky, A. D. (1979). Critique on primal therapy. *The American Journal of Psychotherapy, 33*(1), 119–127. https://doi.org/10.1176/appi.psychotherapy.1979.33.1.119

Index

About the Authors

Barry A. Farber, PhD, is a professor of psychology and education at Teachers College, Columbia University (TC). He received his PhD from Yale University in 1978, joined the clinical psychology faculty at TC the following year, and served as director of clinical training for 24 years. He has varied interests within the area of psychotherapy research, including the nature and consequences of therapists' provision of positive regard, the extent to which patients, therapists, supervisors, and supervisees honestly disclose to each other, and the ways in which individuals construct and evoke mental representations of others, including former therapists and romantic partners, throughout their lives. Previous books include *Secrets and Lies in Psychotherapy, Self-disclosure in Psychotherapy, The Psychotherapy of Carl Rogers,* and *Rock 'n Roll Wisdom.* In addition to his research, writing, and teaching, Dr. Farber recently completed an 8-year term as editor of the *Journal of Clinical Psychology: In Session* and maintains a small private practice of psychotherapy.

Jessica Y. Suzuki, PhD, is a client-centered therapist trained in a relational psychodynamic and experiential approaches. Dr. Suzuki received her PhD from Columbia University Teachers College in 2018, under the research mentorship of Barry Farber, and helmed several research studies on positive regard in psychotherapy throughout her tenure as director of the Positive Regard Lab at TC (2013–2018). She completed her doctoral-level clinical training in hospital-based programs throughout New York City, including the Manhattan VA and Mount Sinai Beth Israel. Dr. Suzuki's early years as a licensed clinician were spent in college mental health positions at Columbia University and New York University. She now operates her own psychotherapy practice in New York City, seeing individuals, couples, and families.

Daisy Ort is a fourth-year doctoral candidate in the Clinical Psychology PhD program at Columbia University Teachers College. Her research experience with the Psychotherapy, Affirmation, & Disclosure Lab began as a master's student at Teachers College in 2013. Prior to beginning her doctoral studies, she worked within New York City's mental health and legal systems conducting research at a criminal justice nonprofit, co-leading weekly support groups at federal jails, and facilitating forensic psychological evaluations for immigration purposes. As a graduate student, she is interested in better understanding relational aspects of psychotherapy across different contexts. Previous research projects assessed the role of informal supervision among psychotherapy trainees and client disclosure in correctional settings. Currently, she and her research team are exploring factors associated with therapists' perceptions of positive regard, as well as clients' experience of teletherapy since the onset of the COVID-19 pandemic.